daily sex

365
POSITIONS
and
ACTIVITIES
for a
YEAR
of
GREAT SEX!

JANE SEDDON

WARNER BOOKS

NEW YORK   BOSTON

This project would have been impossible without my wonderful husband and best friend. Thank you for everything!

This book is intended for use by adults who are informed and want to invigorate and maintain a great sexual relationship. The author is not medically trained, and the reader is reminded that following these guidelines and new ideas is voluntary and at the reader's own discretion. The positions and methodology presented herein are safe and satisfying for most adult men and women; however, every individual is different and you should not undertake any position or technique that is not suitable to your physical condition. You should consult a health care professional with any questions. Certain acts described in this book are illegal in some states and you should be aware of the laws in your state.

Warner Books

Time Warner Book Group
1271 Avenue of the Americas, New York, NY 10020

Printed in the United States of America

ISBN 0-446-69127-5

Book design and text composition by Mada Design, Inc.
Cover design by Brigid Pearson
Cover photo by Barnaby Itall/Photonica

Why Daily Sex?

One day I told a friend of mine that I was writing a book about daily sex. He looked at me in shock and then went on to say that he already works ten hours a day and has an hour-long commute. Now he would have to go home and have sex every night too? My friend clearly needs to change his perspective about sex. Sex is a pleasure, not a punishment. Sex is a chance to share intimate moments with your partner every day. Sex is a chance to indulge the body and mind and feel great. And, unlike many of life's other pleasures, sex does not have fat grams, cost money, or require elaborate equipment.

But daily sex is about more than just physical pleasure. Daily sex also helps form a special bond for a couple. Sex (in a monogamous relationship) is one of the few activities that people participate in exclusively with only one other person. You can love, spend time with, and even share intimate thoughts with parents, kids, friends, and neighbors. But you only have an intimate physical and sexual relationship with your partner. And because of that uniqueness, a special bond exists for the couple. Daily sex helps to nourish and develop that special bond, which in turn will also foster or reinforce love, faithfulness, and loyalty between the couple.

Daily sex will also help each person in the relationship grow stronger and more confident. The variety of sexual positions and activities presented in this book will help identify likes and dislikes both for pleasing someone else and for being pleased themselves. As each person within the relationship grows stronger, the strength of the relationship will also increase. The adage that the whole is better than the sum of the parts is true for relationships. So, as each person in the relationship grows, the relationship itself will also grow and gain strength.

My friend's initial response to the concept of daily sex is not uncommon. Is daily sex for me? Can people really find time for sex every day? Will sex stay interesting even if I do it every day? These are the questions people ask me the most often. The simple answer to all these questions is "yes!" and this book will show you how.

Developing a Great Sexual Relationship

Everyone is capable of enjoying sex every day. However, great sexual relationships typically share some common characteristics that help them succeed. As couples try to improve or expand their physical intimacy, development of these characteristics is important. Some couples may only need to concentrate on one or two items. Other couples might need to work on all the items in the list. All couples that share a willingness to honestly communicate and work together have the tools they need to build a strong and passionate sexual relationship.

First of all, both partners need to be enthusiastic about the sexual relationship. If both people are not truly committed to establishing or maintaining physical intimacy, then a good (or great) sexual relationship will be nearly impossible. Most people lose their sexual desire when their partner is uninterested or reluctant. The best sex occurs when two people are actively and enthusiastically participating in the intercourse.

Couples need to openly and honestly communicate their needs, desires, and goals with regards to physical intimacy. Many of the difficulties that couples face occur when partners have different ideas on what defines a good sexual relationship or even a good sexual position. Maybe there are certain types of foreplay or sexual activities that you particularly like and would like your partner to engage in more frequently. Or conversely, there may be certain activities or positions that you do not like and would prefer not to use. If you don't tell your partner about your preferences and desires, it will be difficult for the relationship to improve. Daily sex will provide couples with ample opportunity to try new things and then discuss what they like, do not like, or would like to change.

Both partners need to display a willingness to try new things. Some of the positions and activities in this book may seem downright silly or senseless, especially for couples that tend to have a very repetitive sex life with only a few positions and variations. Other positions and activities may be perceived as undesirable, but could actually turn out to be very pleasurable and satisfying. By trying the suggested position or activity, you can learn new things about yourself, your partner, and your relationship as a couple. Not all positions and activities are going to please everybody. But even if a couple tries something new and does not like it, they have still engaged in intimacy and learned something new about themselves.

Couples also need to have complete mutual trust and confidence in each other. Because sex is a highly charged emotional activity, participants can feel vulnerable. This vulnerability usually increases when new sexual positions or activities are introduced. Each person needs to know that they have the unconditional support and love from their partner regardless of whether the activity becomes a favorite or is never tried again. Engaging in new and interesting sexual activities in a fully trusting environment is essential to strengthening the emotional bond shared by the couple.

Finally, good sexual relationships exist when each person is willing to please and be pleased. Sex is ultimately about pleasure, both giving it and receiving it. The balance of a relationship will be disrupted if one partner is only interested in giving pleasure or if one partner is only interested in receiving pleasure. It is surprising news for people that only like to give pleasure to find out that by denying their partner a chance to provide pleasure, they are also denying their partner a chance to experience the full intimacy of a sexual relationship. Many people that are currently only interested in receiving pleasure learn that fulfilling a partner's sexual needs adds a totally new dimension to the overall sexual experience.

Finding Time for Sex

Admittedly, one of the biggest obstacles to participating in daily sex is that couples need to allow time for it each day. It's a busy world, and for some people finding the time to take a deep breath every day is a luxury. But remember, sex is pleasurable and fun, and it doesn't have to take a significant amount of time. Making time to engage in a fun and satisfying activity that can potentially improve the overall relationship should be easy to justify. Some nights are perfect for long, passionate romance. Other nights (or maybe most nights?) are more suitable to ten to twenty minutes of love and intimacy. Go to bed fifteen minutes earlier, stay up fifteen minutes later, have sex during the fifteen-minute halftime of the football game on TV. If sex is something you look forward to, you will amaze yourself at the creative ways that can be found for finding time in a busy schedule to include sex. And, as a couple makes sex a daily activity, it becomes a priority for them instead of something that happens when all other items on the to do list have been crossed off.

Of course, there are some legitimate obstacles to having daily sex. A family vacation with a single hotel room is not the appropriate time to make sure that daily sex is a priority! Nor is it possible if one partner is traveling. And, of course, a partner recovering from illness or surgery should not feel pressured into resuming a daily sex life until their health allows it. Although daily sex is suggested and encouraged, common sense and good judgment also need to be exercised.

Sometimes situations can seem like legitimate obstacles, but in reality they just make daily sex more difficult rather than impossible. The thought of having sex after taking care of young children all day or putting in extra hours at work can be very unattractive. The list of reasons and excuses for not participating in daily sex is very long, limited only by our imagination. But how about the thought of your partner holding you and loving you? Instead of focusing on the negative aspects of the situation, think about the positive feeling you get from great sex and connecting intimately with your partner. Surprisingly, what typically happens when a couple goes ahead with daily sex even on days where one of them is tired is that the sexual act becomes a highlight of the day. Oftentimes it's even therapeutic. On days like this where sex seems undesirable, the hardest part is getting started. Once the couple becomes involved in the activity, many of the day's stresses can be temporarily forgotten.

Keeping Sex Interesting

Daily sex is about more than just frequency; it's also about having *great* sex. So although using the same position every day qualifies as daily sex, it would not necessarily qualify as great sex. In fact, using the same position day after day would turn sex into a monotonous chore. For sex to stay fun, it needs to stay interesting. The easiest way to keep it interesting is variety, variety, variety.

Variety comes in many different ways. First of all, this book includes several different forms of sex. Each month you'll find positions for sexual intercourse, oral sex, and manual sex. Then there is variety within each type of sex. There are an extraordinary number of different positions and techniques to try. You need to explore your partner's entire body to locate all their erogenous zones.

Each month also includes activities designed to add some zest to your love life. Some of the activities enhance the sexual act itself; others focus on the seduction and foreplay leading up to sex. Although seduction and foreplay are not the main focus of this book, they are still important to the overall sexual experience. Good foreplay will enhance the sexual positions, techniques, and activities you try.

The Physical and Emotional Aspects of Sex

Sex is an activity that is both physically and emotionally intense. Altering either aspect will change the overall sensations experienced. The greatest physical position in the world is not very satisfying when the people involved are not in the mood for sex. Conversely, even the standard missionary position can be very arousing, stimulating, and highly pleasing when the couple is emotionally bonding with each other.

All of the intercourse positions presented in this book are physically unique. In some cases, the differences between the positions are very obvious. Some have the man on top; others have the woman on top. The couple can be lying down, sitting, standing, or kneeling. Even if the person is lying down, they can have their head and shoulders elevated by resting on their elbows or their legs could be hanging over the edge of the bed. When the woman is on top, she can be facing her partner's head or his feet.

Other differences, such as the placement of each person's legs, are much more subtle. When a woman lies on her back with her legs basically straight in front of her, her partner's access to her vagina is more restricted than when the woman's legs are spread wide open or wrapped around her partner's waist. This subtle difference causes a significant change in the depth of penetration. Differences are also felt when the woman is on top and leans forward or backward. When men are on the bottom or sitting, they will find that when they change the position of their legs, it affects their ability to thrust. This is an important issue for some men, but not for everyone.

Physical changes to the position can impact the depth, angle, and tightness of the penetration. Each individual decides whether the change is an improvement. Many women rave about positions where the penis is at an angle that stimulates their G-spot. Other women are still not convinced the G-spot actually exists. Some positions are very tight, but not very deep. Each couple needs to be attentive to both the large and small variations because both can cause considerable changes to the overall enjoyment.

The Emotional Aspects of Sex

A single physical intercourse position can be experienced many different ways depending on each person's mood and the ambience of the environment. So, although this book includes 365 different physical positions, there is, additionally, a multitude of ways of trying each one. We'll use the Back Seat Special (Month 1, Day 30) as an example.

This position can be a very romantic, loving, tender expression of feelings. Romantic sex, typically conducted at a slower pace, is usually more time-consuming than other types of sex. Romantic sex strongly addresses the emotional aspects of sex with lots of kissing, cuddling, caressing, and eye contact. When romantically using the Back Seat Special, the couple can take advantage of being face-to-face by whispering compliments and expressions of love to each other. Of course, the overall ambience of the situation and the environment also contribute to the degree of romance the couple will experience. Candles, soft music, and a good massage are just a few ways to help generate romance.

Humorous or playful sex is much more light-hearted, but will strengthen a relationship by providing couples with a chance to share a good laugh and have some fun. Humorous sex, sometimes the best type of sex, can be therapeutic at the end of a difficult and stressful day. Some activities, such as wearing sunglasses or shoes during intercourse, help encourage a playful environment. Other times, humorous sex can occur spontaneously. Any couple that has tried a tricky new position has probably experienced a good laugh as they try to work out where all the arms and legs are supposed to go. While using the Back Seat Special, laugh and have fun with your partner. Playfully tease each other. Ladies, while your partner is kissing you, gently bite down and lock his tongue between your teeth.

Clandestine sex — sex at an unusual location or time — is a great way for couples to feel close by sharing a secret. An example of clandestine sex is a quickie in the bathroom while the kids are in the family room watching television. Other examples are having sex outside during the day, a quickie just before going out to a formal party, or using the Back Seat Special in the taxi on the way to your in-laws' house. For many couples, the excitement of doing something just a little bit naughty and secretive helps forge a special bond.

Experimental sex, agreeing as a couple to try new sexual activities, promotes a sense of teamwork and cooperation. Many of the activities suggested in this book are designed to help each person learn more about their partner. Even after many years of marriage, it's amazing the amount of new information we can still learn about our mate. While using the Back Seat Special, play around with a vibrator. Although you're sitting pretty close together, see what happens when you wedge the vibrator between the two of you. Guys, you can reach behind your partner and see what she thinks about some anal stimulation. Experimental sex can result in many new intercourse variations that can transform good sex into great sex.

Functional sex is the type of sex that occurs at all other times. In a perfect world, sexual intercourse would always be deeply moving and highly exciting. In reality, there are times when sex is routine. (Of course, if sexual intercourse was always highly romantic or humorous, this would also become routine.) Everyday, ordinary, routine sex is a normal part of life. Using the Back Seat Special on the couch during the five-minute commercial break is functional sex. It's called functional sex because it works. It's still fun, pleasurable, and satisfying, and should still be considered a wonderful expression of love.

How to Use This Book

This book contains a year's worth of sexual activities divided into twelve thirty-day chapters. Although the chronological year begins on January 1, your sexual year can start on any day of any month.

Once the commitment to daily sex has been made, couples should start with the first day of the first month, regardless of the actual chronological date. An extra chapter has been included at the end of the book with extra positions to be used during months with thirty-one days.

During some months, it might be necessary to adjust the suggested calendar to fit particular circumstances. For example, some couples might find that the more time-consuming activities are better suited for weekend nights. A couple might also agree that certain activities will not occur during a woman's menstrual cycle. Both partners need to be flexible and keep an open mind to all aspects of the sexual relationship.

Couples that find it impossible or undesirable to engage in daily sex will, obviously, not be able to finish a thirty-day calendar in thirty days. When a day (or more) is skipped, the position or activity suggested on the missed day should be used when daily sex resumes. Some couples will find that it takes eighteen months to two years to finish a year's worth of positions. There is nothing wrong with that.

Very few people will like everything that they try in the book. Refrain from eliminating positions or activities from the calendar simply because they are new, different, or make a person feel self-conscious. One of the benefits of daily sex is that everyone gets to learn more about themselves and their partners. You'll never learn what you like if you never try anything new. Of course, if you try a certain type of position several times and find that it's undesirable, the remaining positions of this type can be skipped. For example, some men will find that it's

uncomfortable to kneel with their legs completely bent. Others might dislike positions where the penetration results in an angle that is contrary to how their penis naturally hangs.

The description for each position includes a rating scale. I suggest that you use it, especially to mark positions that you particularly like or don't like. Although you might think you can remember every great position you try, odds are that you won't. Of course, trying them all again to find your favorites is not necessarily a bad thing either!

Cautions

Sexual intercourse should always be a consensual act. Even if both partners have agreed to daily sex, if one person says no on a particular day, then the partner needs to be respectful of their wishes. Days may exist when the reason one person does not want to have daily sex looks like an excuse to the other person. If this happens frequently, the couple needs to reexamine their commitment to daily sex.

The positions and activities suggested in this book are intended to increase the pleasure derived from physical intimacy. However, if one of the positions or activities inadvertently causes pain or discomfort, then the position or activity should be stopped. In some cases, a minor modification to the position or activity will eliminate the problem.

1 MONTH 1

Day 1. Sideswiped

Day 2. Give the Dog a Bone

Day 3. The Necklace

Day 4. Kissing Booth

Day 5. Feather in Your...Cap?

Day 6. Cream with Your Coffee?

Day 7. Pole Position

Day 8. Head-on Collision

Day 9. Poking Fun

Day 10. Splitting at the Seams

Day 11. Blind Leading the Blind

Day 12. X Marks the Spot

Day 13. Sunny and 90 Degrees

Day 14. Beat Around the Bush

Day 15. Popsicle

Day 16. Feel the Magic

Day 17. Seeing Stars

Day 18. Sidesaddle

Day 19. Dinner for Two

Day 20. Snake in the Grass

Day 21. Slippery When Wet

Day 22. Bounty Hunter

Day 23. Turn Up the Heat

Day 24. Cat Got Your Tongue?

Day 25. Attached at the Hips

Day 26. Sandman's Surprise

Day 27. Stirrups

Day 28. Head Over Heels

Day 29. In Over My Head

Day 30. Back Seat Special

Sideswiped

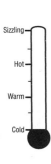

Sizzling

Hot

Warm

Cold

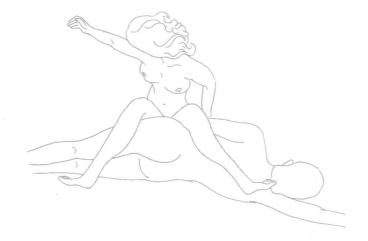

Let's start the year with a position that provides great sideways penetration. The man lies on his side with his legs together. Ladies, you'll have to do most of the work to achieve penetration with this one. Start by sitting perpendicular to the man and putting your legs over his hips. Then, using one hand behind you to support your weight and one hand to guide his penis, move your bottom as close to the man as possible. Lift or lower your hips as needed until the height and angle of your vagina allows your lover's penis to slide right in. Now that you've done your part, lie back and start enjoying.

Guys, you'll be responsible for the thrusting. With the woman's clitoris so easily accessible in this position, manual stimulation is a must! The woman can do this herself, but it's even better when you guys do it for her. Use a side-to-side motion with your fingertips and time your thrusts to match the pace. Ladies, increase the intensity a bit by massaging your breasts and nipples. It feels great, and men just love to watch! With a little luck and some practice, this position will be a great opportunity for simultaneous orgasms!

Give the Dog a Bone

Month 1
Day 2

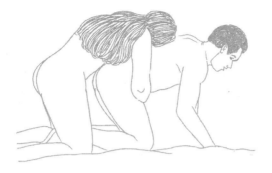

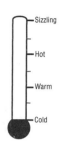

Sizzling

Hot

Warm

Cold

This is a nonintercourse position in which the woman masturbates the man. So ladies, get ready to please your guy!

Both the man and the woman assume the traditional doggy-style stance. But this position is a little unusual because the man is in front of the woman instead of behind her. Ladies, wrap your arm around your partner's waist and firmly grasp the shaft of his penis. And certainly don't limit yourself to just penile stimulation. Excite him with your breasts by pressing them into his back or grazing his back with your nipples. Lean forward and kiss him on his ears and the back of his neck. Whisper into his ear how much you love him. Guys, as your partner experiments with various ways of stimulating you, let her know which ones you find the most exciting. It enhances the pleasure for you, and she'll appreciate the feedback.

Be sure to include yourself in the fun, gals. While keeping one hand on the man's penis, use your other hand to masturbate yourself. Not only is it a great physical stimulation for you, it's also a real turn-on for your guy. Or try rubbing your clitoris up against the man's buttocks or hips while your arm is around his waist. This keeps both your hands free to stimulate him. As he becomes more and more aroused, increase the intensity and tempo as your hand moves up and down his penis, until he reaches orgasm.

The Necklace

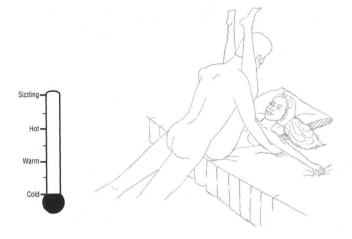

Sizzling—

Hot—

Warm—

Cold—

It's not made of gold, but the human necklace the man wears in this position feels much better and is far more valuable.

In order for the man to achieve penetration, the woman needs to lie on her back with her pelvis and hips as close to the edge of the bed as possible, with her legs bent and her feet on the floor. The man will penetrate the woman by leaning up against the bed at an angle where his penis can be guided into the woman's vagina. If need be, the man should lift his lover's buttocks and move

her closer. To help support his weight, the man needs to have his hands on either side of the woman's shoulders and his arms should be straight.

Once penetration has occurred, the woman needs to move her legs up to the man's shoulders. This is a step that is impossible to do without coordination between the couple. The woman lifts one foot off the floor and moves it toward the man's shoulder, while the man moves his arm out of the way. This, of course, needs to happen for each leg. This might sound a little

tricky, but it's actually not that difficult and definitely worth the extra effort.

Now the fun stuff can start!

Ladies, if clitoral stimulation helps you to orgasm during intercourse, then you're going to like this because the man's pelvis is resting right up against you. Wiggle your hips and bottom around until you've found a sensitive spot that gets stimulated each time he thrusts. For even stronger stimulation, use your hands to press down on his buttocks and increase the pressure of his pelvis on your clitoris. Guys, with penetration this deep and your lover grabbing hold of you, you'll need to pace yourself so that both of you will have an opportunity to orgasm!

Kissing Booth

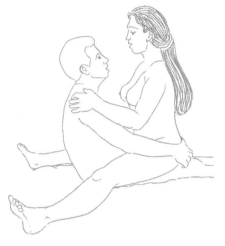

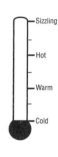

If you like to kiss and cuddle, then this position is fantastic!

It's also a very simple position to achieve. The man sits on the bed with his legs straight in front of him. The woman sits on the man's lap, facing her partner, with her legs spread open in front of her. Ladies, the closer you sit and the wider you spread your legs, the deeper the penetration. So inch up as close as you can get and open wide!

This position is great for a night when the mood is tender and loving and the emphasis is on kissing. Many couples who have been together for a while don't even bother with kissing anymore. So start with slow, shallow kisses to the face and neck. Look each other in the eyes. Touch your lover's face and hair. Nibble on their ears. Pretend it's the first time the two of you have met and you're exploring each other for the first time. Gradually increase the intensity until the two of you are passionately and deeply tongue to tonsils!

Deep thrusting needs to accompany the deep kissing. The best way to accomplish this is for the man and woman to work together. Ladies, lift and lower your hips up and down your partner's penis. Clench your vaginal muscles to keep the penetration tight. Guys, lift and lower your hips synchronously with your partner. As her hips come down, your hips go up. Keep your hips and lips locked together until both of you have orgasmed.

Feather in Your...Cap?

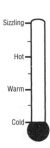

Sizzling

Hot

Warm

Cold

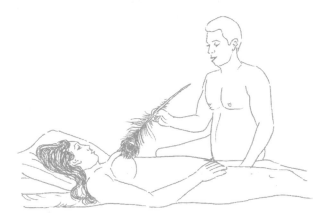

You'll need a clean feather for this activity. They are cheap and easy to find at any craft or discount store.

Guys, this is a manual stimulation activity with a delicate touch. Use the feather to tickle and stimulate your lover. The touch is so light and soft that it drives women wild. Start with the face and neck and slowly move down your lover's body. Rub the feather under her chin. Tickle her on the ear. Run the feather from her neck down to her breasts. Brush it lightly against her nipples. Swish the feather from side to side as you lightly tickle her tummy. Just when she thinks you'll be getting to the most exciting bits, switch to her feet and start working your way back up. Give attention to her feet, her ankles, her calves, behind her knees, and the insides of her thighs. Slowly and gently work your way to her hips and pelvis. Use the feather to stimulate your lover's genitals. Rub the feather around the outside of her vagina. Tickle the sensitive perineum. Glide it back and forth across her clitoris.

Ladies, enjoy the soft, delicate sensation of the feather against your skin. When you start experiencing sensory overload, let your partner know it's time to switch from the feather to his fingers. Guys, rub your fingers back and forth across your lover's clitoris. Gradually increase the tempo until she reaches her peak.

Cream with Your Coffee?

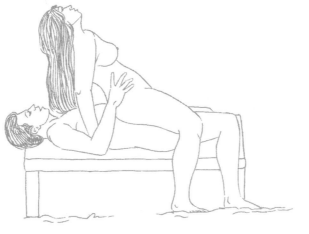

Sizzling

Hot

Warm

Cold

Clear the coffee table for this one because what a difference the angle of the legs can make! This position looks similar to many other positions where the man is lying on his back and the woman sits on top of him. But what makes this position interesting and unique is that instead of having their legs flat on the bed, both the man and the woman have their legs straddling a piece of furniture. And coffee tables work great for this! The downward pull of the leg muscles combined with the woman leaning backward result in a wonderfully snug and deep penetration at an unusual angle.

Guys, take advantage of having your feet on the floor. The extra leverage allows for very strong and deep thrusting.

Ladies, try supporting your weight by leaning back on just one arm. Use your free hand to reach down between your guy's legs and start massaging his testicles. You'll have cream for your coffee in no time!

Pole Position

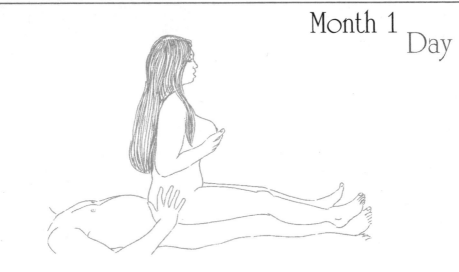

Sizzling —
Hot —
Warm —
Cold —

Women who like to take control are going to love this position because they are definitely in the driver's seat.

Guys, lie on your back with your legs straight out in front of you. Ladies, sit on top of the man facing the man's feet. Start with your legs spread open. This allows you to reach between your legs to grasp your man's penis and guide it to the proper spot for insertion. Once penetration has occurred, put your legs together and rest them on the man's legs. For optimum tightness, close your legs as far as possible without causing discomfort or disrupting penetration.

Men, relax and enjoy being a passenger on this one! Feel free to grab your partner's buttocks to help her maneuver herself around and find the best angle. Or better yet, gently stroke her back and enjoy the view.

Start your engine, ladies! You get to control the angle, depth, and tempo of the thrusting. Slow and easy or hard and fast — women, you choose the pace tonight.

Head-on Collision

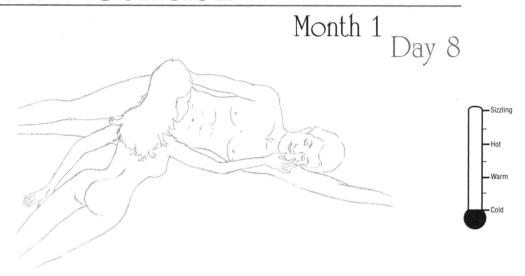

Sizzling

Hot

Warm

Cold

Check your insurance coverage because this collision is sure to knock you out!

The man lies comfortably on his side. Some men find it convenient to have a wall behind them to lean against. Some men like to keep both legs straight; others like to have one leg bent. Do whatever feels right for you.

The woman lies perpendicular to the man, usually on her stomach.

Ideally, she will be just out of the man's reach — leaving him powerless to do anything but watch and enjoy.

Ladies, using one hand on his shaft for support, start to gently lick around the head of the man's penis. Your mouth is warm and moist and he wants to be in it, but tease him for a little while with just some tongue action. Use your other hand to caress his face and chest

or massage his testicles. Finally, put his penis in your mouth and give him his total pleasure. While keeping him in your mouth, run your tongue around the head and up and down the shaft. Because you are lying sideways to him, the angle of your mouth will be completely different from many of the other fellatio positions. Drive him wild!

Poking Fun

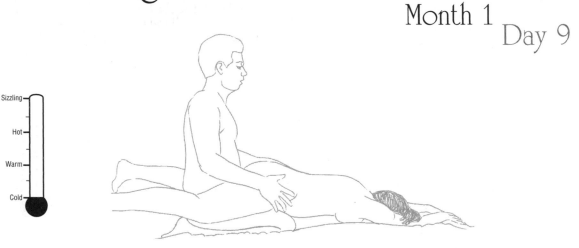

Sizzling
Hot
Warm
Cold

For some of you guys, the most difficult part of this position will be kneeling with your legs folded completely underneath you. Relax your leg muscles and bend your knees. Once you get started, that stiffness in your legs will be replaced by a more intense and pleasurable stiffness somewhere else!

Once the man is successfully kneeling, the woman straddles him, facing the same direction he is facing. Help her out here, guys. Use your hands on her buttocks to slowly pull her backward and help guide her onto your penis. Following penetration, the woman should lean all the way forward with her arms flat against the bed.

Guys, for deeper penetration, hold your lover's buttocks while you're thrusting. Move her up and down the shaft of your penis. This is also a great position for you to actually see your penis sliding in and out of your lover's vagina. Very, very erotic! Massage, tickle, and explore your lover's bottom. With her permission, use a finger and give her some anal penetration. It'll make her toes tingle!

Splitting at the Seams

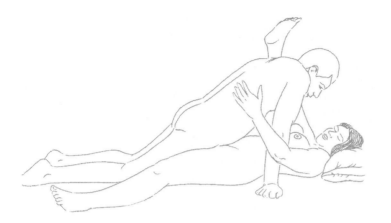

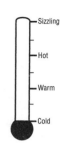

This variation of the standard missionary position looks like it's been designed for a gymnast. But fear not. It's much easier than it appears!

The woman lies on her back with one leg between the man's legs. The woman's other leg goes in front of the man's arm and rests on his shoulder or neck. Are you afraid you can't stretch like this? Don't worry! I have never in my life been able to do a split but can easily handle this position.

Men, with your pelvis resting on the woman's clitoris, this is a great position for helping her achieve orgasm. Move your hips around a bit until you feel her responding to your thrusts. Then you'll know you've found a good spot! Also, take advantage of her leg on your shoulder. Massage her foot and kiss her ankle. Women love this!

Blind Leading the Blind

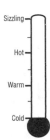

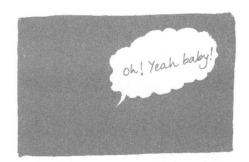

For this activity, you'll have intercourse in complete darkness. The first challenge is to find a spot that is completely dark because "completely dark" is more than just a room with no lights on. It's a place where you can't even see your hand in front of your face. So if the room you plan to use has windows, they need to be covered with something that totally blocks any light from outside. A rolled-up towel is a great way to stop light from entering a room from under the door. The best places for this activity (besides a cave) are bathrooms, large closets, pantries, and media rooms. If it's not possible to find a completely dark room, both the man and the woman should wear blindfolds.

Once an appropriate location has been found, the couple can proceed to engage in their normal foreplay activities and choose any intercourse position they want. If the room is truly completely black, the couple will not be able to see each other at all. The sensory deprivation of losing sight accentuates the other senses, particularly the sense of touch.

The best part of this activity is that the couple will have to explore each other with just their hands in order to get all the right body parts into the right places. Even simple positions can become tricky when you can't see what you're doing. The loss of sight will heighten the pleasure, and sometimes the humor.

X Marks the Spot

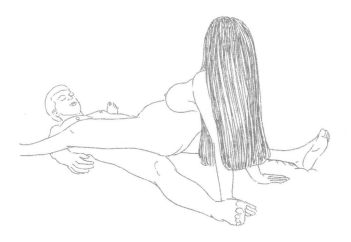

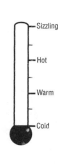

Traditionally used on pirates' maps to mark buried treasure, the X created when you have your treasure buried in this position is definitely worth remembering!

For this position, the man is lying on his back with his legs spread wide open. The woman sits on the man, facing him, with her legs also spread wide open. Then, to make the penetration especially tight, the woman leans backward onto her arms.

Ladies, this is a wonderful position for you to do the thrusting. With your arms holding most of your weight, your hips have a lot of freedom to move around. Don't limit yourself to just thrusting forward and backward. Move your hips from side to side. Grind them around in a circle. Don't be surprised if your man grabs your buttocks and holds you still while he suddenly discovers the treasure!

Sunny and 90 Degrees

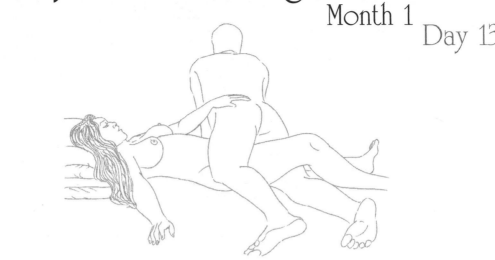

Sizzling

Hot

Warm

Cold

This position can be a little tricky to get started, but it's definitely worth the effort. The woman lies on her back with one leg between the man's legs. The man assumes a missionary position, but at a 90 degree angle to the woman. Penetration can be a little challenging at first. Because the man is lying sideways, his penis will be pointing to the side too. Ladies, you need to gently guide his penis into your vagina. But be careful! Bending his penis to achieve penetration is not a sexual stimulant for most men!

An alternative method of achieving this position is to start in the standard missionary position. The man can then rotate his hands and body to the side while maintaining penetration.

Women will find that this position will hit spots inside of them that they didn't even know existed. Most intercourse positions stimulate either the back or front wall of the vagina. In this case, the penis is actually pushing to the side instead.

Ladies, how can anyone resist a man's cute buns? Tickle, tease, spank, and please. His buttocks are right there in front of you. Have a great time!

Beat Around the Bush

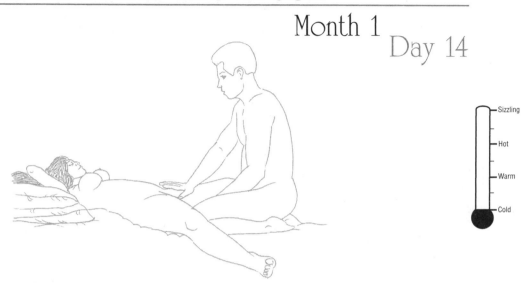

Sizzling

Hot

Warm

Cold

Better yet, rub gently, but firmly, around the bush! Guys, this is a chance to make the woman in your life wiggle and squirm with pleasure.

Ladies, your only requirement is to lie comfortably on your back and enjoy, enjoy, enjoy!

The man should spread apart the woman's legs and kneel between them. Start slowly by just rubbing her pubic hair and tickling the tops of her thighs with your fingers. Gradually increase the pressure and start moving closer to the clitoris. Most women will require direct clitoral stimulation to orgasm, but don't rush there right away. Rub the areas around the clitoris, and tease her by briefly rubbing directly on the clitoris as you move from one side to the other. This will drive her crazy. Finally, bring her to orgasm by rubbing back and forth directly on the clitoris. Move your fingers around a bit until you find the most sensitive spot. And guys, there is no reason to leave yourself out of the fun. You can use your other hand to masturbate yourself. However, your primary focus should be pleasing the woman until she comes. After that, bring yourself to orgasm too.

Popsicle

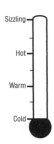

Sizzling —

Hot —

Warm —

Cold —

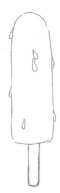

Ladies, put some ice cubes in a glass because you're going to show your man just how great frigid can be!

Just before inserting your lover's penis head into your mouth, suck on an ice cube for five to ten seconds, or until your mouth feels very cold. Remove the ice cube, and then immediately close your mouth around the penis head and start performing fellatio. The shock of your cold, wet mouth on his warm, dry penis will stimulate nerve endings in the head of his penis that he didn't even know existed. As your mouth warms up, suck on the ice cube and then suck on his penis again. The sensation is so incredibly intense that guys will feel tingly all the way to their toes.

Advanced Popsicle eating: If the ice cubes are small, keep one ice cube in your mouth while simultaneously sucking and licking the penis head. Move the ice cube around with your tongue so that it briefly comes in direct contact with the penis. This little trick extends the period of time the mouth is cold and greatly intensifies the overall experience.

Feel the Magic

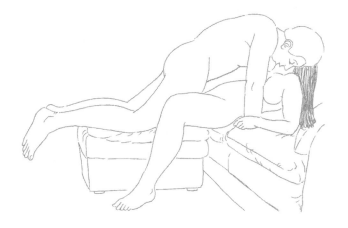

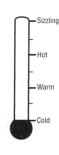

Guys, use your magic wand properly, and you'll both feel the magic!

This position requires a piece of furniture that is narrow enough for the woman to straddle, but wide enough for the man to kneel on. It's important that the woman be able to straddle the piece of furniture and not just have her legs opened wide. Having her legs bent toward the floor creates a downward angle that pulls down on the vaginal muscles and creates a tight penetration. An ottoman pushed against a sofa works great for this.

The woman straddles the ottoman, but does not lie flat on her back. She keeps her arms bent underneath her so that her shoulders are elevated and her weight is on her elbows. The man kneels down between the woman's legs. Guys, as you lean forward, use one of your hands to guide your penis into your lover's vagina. Once you've penetrated, put both of your hands next to your partner's arms so that you can rest your weight on your wrists. If the woman's feet reach the floor, she can push off and help with the thrusting. Most of the thrusting, however, will be done by the man.

Guys, finish the magic potion by kissing your lover's face and neck. "Accidentally" brush your chest against her nipples. She'll be spellbound!

Seeing Stars

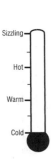

Sizzling

Hot

Warm

Cold

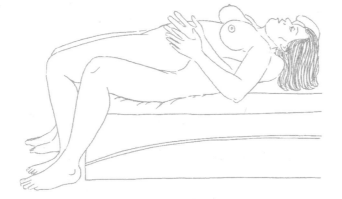

This position is good in the bedroom, but great outside on the picnic table as well! Stargazing will never be the same again.

The man lies on his back with his legs over the edge of the bed or table. If you're doing this outside and your feet don't touch the ground, put your feet on the picnic bench. You'll need the leverage for thrusting.

Women, the easiest way to get penetration for this position is to start by sitting on your partner's lap facing away from him. Your legs should be outside your partner's legs. Once his penis is inside, carefully lift your legs and move them to the inside of his legs. Finally, lean backward all the way to your partner's chest. With your legs close together, this is a nice snug fit that many of you will find very stimulating to your vaginal muscles.

Guys, put your arms around your lover and hold her tight. Women love how comfortable and secure it feels to be in their man's strong embrace. Massage her breasts, enjoying the full access you get because she's lying on her back. Ladies, your legs are together pretty close, but you should be able to get your fingers in there for some manual clitoral stimulation.

Even on a cloudy night, this position will have you seeing stars!

Sidesaddle

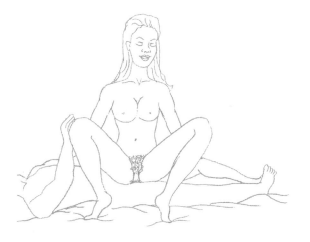

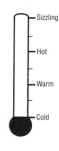

Sizzling

Hot

Warm

Cold

Before women wore pants, they had to ride horses sidesaddle so that they would look ladylike and to keep their skirts looking proper. But riding the horse sidesaddle in this position doesn't require skirts or pants. And ladylike behavior is optional too!

The man lies on his back with his legs straight in front of him. The woman sits sideways on the man. For deep penetration, her legs should be spread open and completely bent at the knees. Gals, you'll be doing most of the thrusting on this one.

Sideways penetration is a unique sensation that must be experienced to be understood. The vaginal walls around the penis feel completely different than when the woman is facing forward or backward. For some women, the ever-elusive G-spot is stimulated from a sideways position. I wonder if the women riding sidesaddle in the olden days ever experienced that!

Dinner for Two

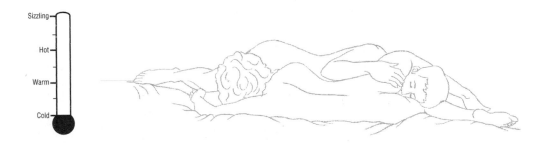

Sizzling
Hot
Warm
Cold

Soixante-neuf — the French word for 69. This is a classic oral sex position that dates back at least as far as the *Kama Sutra*.

The man and woman lie side to side with their heads on opposite ends. The woman performs fellatio on the man while, at the same time, the man is performing cunnilingus on the woman.

Sounds so simple, but this position is very steamy! It's difficult to concentrate on what your mouth is doing, when the other person's mouth is making you feel sooo good! Use your hands to grasp the other person's buttocks. This will prevent them from wiggling away as they squirm in pleasure.

Ladies, be careful not to accidentally bite! Climaxing while the man's penis is in your mouth can lead to some very unpleasant mishaps. Since it's virtually impossible to fully enjoy your orgasm and concentrate on what your mouth is doing, remove the man's penis from your mouth when your orgasm is near. The slight interruption in fellatio is well worth it!

Snake in the Grass

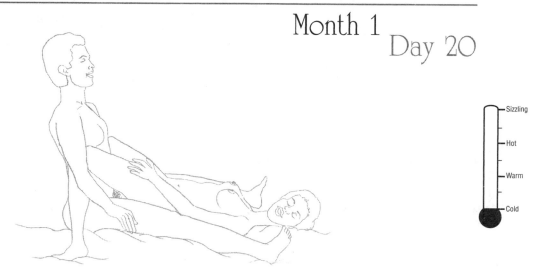

Sizzling

Hot

Warm

Cold

I don't think this is what the Roman poet Virgil had in mind when he warned about a snake in the grass. This snake isn't evil and it's certainly not a cold-blooded reptile!

The man sits with his legs spread open. The woman lies on her back between the man's legs. The woman's legs are bent over the man's thighs with her feet pressed up close to the man's hips. Women, scoot your hips and pelvis as far forward as possible for the deepest penetration.

Okay, guys, this one is a no-brainer. Your lover is lying in front of you with her legs spread wide open. I don't think I need to tell you what a great opportunity this is for clitoral stimulation! Focus directly on the clitoris and the small area around it. As your lover becomes more aroused, you will feel her clitoris swelling beneath your fingers. As you bring her to her peak, you'll love the way she thrusts her hips forward as she orgasms!

Slippery When Wet

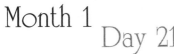

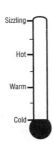

Sizzling

Hot

Warm

Cold

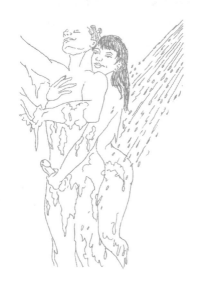

Ladies, this is a water activity where you will manually stimulate your man's penis with your hands. It can very easily be done in the bathtub or the shower, so pick the location and get started. In theory, this activity could be done with just the man in the bathtub or shower. But it's a lot more fun when both of you are getting wet! So get in the shower or bathtub together to fully enjoy this one.

Ever notice how slippery the skin gets when it's wet?

Your wet hand. His wet penis. Stroking him up and down his shaft is so smooth and easy! You'll need to take this one slow to keep him from climaxing too soon. Alternate between masturbating the shaft and paying attention to other areas. Massage his testicles. Then focus again on stroking the shaft. Use one hand to just stimulate the head of the penis very delicately with your fingertips. Then focus again on stroking the shaft. Rub the head of his

penis on your soft silky skin. Then focus again on stroking the shaft. When he's ready to climax, firmly hold the base of his penis while stroking him.

For the more adventurous types, use a swimming pool for this activity. Ladies, slip your hand up into his shorts and move it up and down the shaft until he reaches orgasm. If you do this quietly, nobody else even needs to know what's happening!

Bounty Hunter

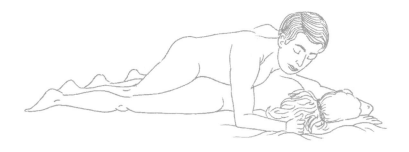

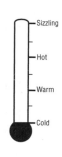

You've missed your court appearance and now he's coming to get you. Or, maybe, he'll be coming when he gets you. With the full body press of this position, no handcuffs will be needed to keep you from running.

This is a rear-entry position where both people are basically lying flat. The easiest way to perform this position is for both to start out in the standard hands-and-knees doggy-style position. Then slowly extend your legs backward and lower your entire upper body to the bed. Caution: If this is not done as a coordinated effort, it will be impossible to maintain penetration! Guys, especially big guys, try to keep some of your weight on your legs and arms. Struggling to take a breath is not a turn-on for most women!

Although this position does not provide much opportunity to use your hands, the biggest benefit of this position is the amount of skin-to-skin contact. You can't get much closer than this! The angle and tightness of penetration also frequently results in enough stimulation to the woman's G-spot to result in orgasm.

Turn Up the Heat

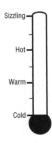

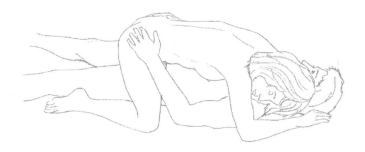

This is a fairly tame woman-on-top position that can range from warm to very hot. So get ready to turn up the heat!

The man lies on his back with his legs straight out in front of him. The woman climbs on top with her legs completely bent and straddling the man.

Ladies, you get to supply the heat. After penetration has occurred, lean forward toward your partner's face. This minor movement significantly changes the angle of penetration. A man's penis naturally points upward when erect, so by leaning forward, you're providing him with the path of least resistance. Also, spread your legs wide enough so that your pubic bone is right up to the man's hips. The deep, smooth, hot penetration is sure to get his temperature rising.

Guys, use your arms and hands to hold your lover close. Pull her face to yours and indulge in some deep kissing. Whisper in her ear how hot you are for her. Enjoy the heat wave while it lasts!

Cat Got Your Tongue?

Month 1
Day 24

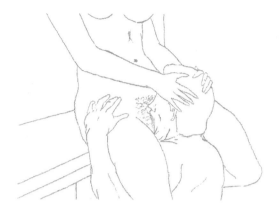

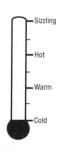

Me-ow! When this pussycat gets your tongue, she'll be purring!

This is a cunnilingus position, ladies, so take a seat, spread your legs nice and wide, and relax!

Guys, the rest is up to you. Start by kneeling on the floor between the woman's legs. Gently open them wider if you need more room. Use your hands to pull her hips up close to the edge of the chair to give you the best angle.

Slowly, but firmly, start licking the area around her clitoris. Move your tongue around randomly looking for the most sensitive spots. When you feel your lover's hips start moving around, you'll know you've found one! Keep your hands on her hips to help hold her in place. She wants to move around, but being held down will actually increase her level of pleasure. Glide your tongue back and forth over your lover's clitoris making each movement a little firmer and quicker as her arousal increases. Relax your hands as she gets ready to orgasm to allow her hips to thrust with the pleasure.

Attached at the Hips

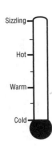

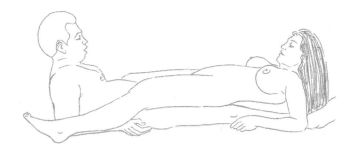

This position is similar to the position used in Day 12 of this month, but what a difference a few minor changes make!

Guys, in this position, you have your legs together straight in front of you. You also need to bend your arms and raise your upper body so that your weight rests on your elbows. Ladies, you're on top again for this position so sit on your man with your legs spread wide open. Then, lean backward with your arms straight behind you.

The biggest benefit with this position, guys, is that your upper body is elevated. First of all, this lets you watch the penetration. Seeing your lover sliding up and down your penis will make your hair tingle. Oh, so nice! Having your upper body raised also makes manually stimulating your partner much easier. Rest your weight on one elbow. Use your other hand to masturbate her clitoris. As the intensity increases, her thrusting will become quicker and deeper until both of you climax.

Sandman's Surprise

Month 1
Day 26

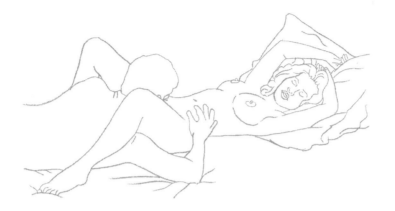

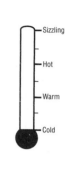

Guys, drinks lots of coffee all day because this activity requires you to be awake while your lover is asleep. Some of you will find this to be pretty easy. Others, especially those with a lover who is a light sleeper, might find this activity impossible.

This activity starts after the woman has fallen soundly asleep. Gently and slowly move your sleeping lover's legs so they are spread open wide enough for you to get between them with your face. Move them as little as possible to avoid accidentally waking her. Lower your mouth onto her clitoris and use your tongue to stimulate her. No need to start slow on this one. You want her to be fully aroused as soon as she wakes up. For most women, this will be fairly quickly after the cunnilingus has started. But don't let this stop you. Continue to rub your tongue back and forth until she orgasms.

Ladies, if you've never woken up to being sexually stimulated, you are in for a huge treat! It is extremely erotic to wake up to the warm, tingly sensation of oral sex!

Stirrups

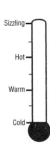

Sizzling

Hot

Warm

Cold

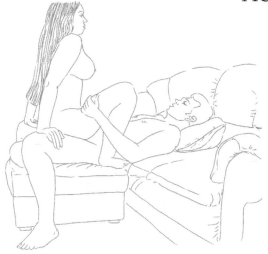

Put your feet in the stirrups and ride this horse to the finish line!

You'll need a thin piece of furniture for this position. A narrow bed or an ottoman pushed up next to the couch work great. The man lies on his back with his legs straddling the ottoman. For the strongest thrusting, his feet should be on the floor. The woman sits facing the man with her legs bent completely up to her chest as if she is squatting. For the best penetration, view, and clitoral access, her thighs should be spread open.

Ladies, this position is great because the guy is doing the thrusting and both of your hands are free! Time to give your man a little treat — a close-up view of you masturbating. For many women, being watched while they masturbate sparks a little extra arousal. The guy certainly feels that extra spark while he's watching you! And, to really send him flying, use your other hand to reach down behind you between his legs and massage his testicles. Having your feet in the stirrups has never felt this good before!

Head Over Heels

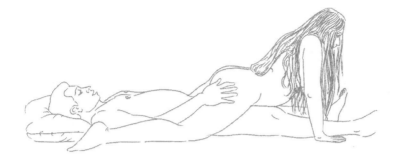

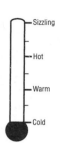

Sizzling

Hot

Warm

Cold

Sometimes it's more than just an expression!

The man lies on his back with his legs straight in front of him. The woman straddles the man with her head toward the man's feet. Using your hands to support your weight, slowly lower yourself onto the man's penis. Adjust the height and angle of your hips to maximize a deep, smooth penetration.

Guys, leave your contacts in because this position has a view worth seeing. As the woman moves forward and backward thrusting, you can see your penis sliding in and out of her vagina. Put your hand around the base of your penis. It intensifies the physical sensation you feel on each thrust, and also feels great each time the woman's warm, moist vulva pushes into your hand. You'll be head over heels in love with this position in no time!

In Over My Head

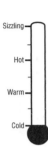

Sizzling

Hot

Warm

Cold

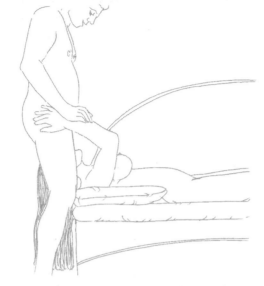

This fellatio position has so many options, it's guaranteed to satisfy everyone!

The woman lies on the bed with her head at the edge. Guys, stand next to the bed and straddle your partner's head with your body facing the bed. Lean forward and rest your weight on the bed for balance. Women, if you have a tall lover, you might need a pillow under your head and neck for some added height.

Ladies, after you've inserted the man's penis into your mouth, you've got two free hands and a lot of choices. Use one hand to grip the base of the man's penis or massage his testicles while performing fellatio. Use the other hand to manually stimulate your clitoris. Spread your legs open wide. Men love to watch women masturbate, and this position gives him a front row seat!

Guys, stroke and caress your lover's breasts and stomach while she masturbates. Or if watching is not enough, join in. When you lean forward just a bit, you can use your hands to manually stimulate her clitoris. When you lean forward a lot, you can bend your head all the way down and perform cunnilingus! Your lover will be very appreciative of the extra attention!

Experiment with the different options, find the ones that work best for you — and ENJOY!

Back Seat Special

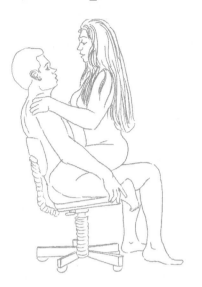

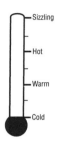

Use your imagination, because this position is not limited to a chair. This is a very versatile position that is particularly useful in the back seat of a car — or a taxi!

The man sits in the chair with his knees bent and his feet on the floor. The woman sits on the man's lap in the direction of the man's face. The woman's legs are on either side of the man's thighs and are bent completely at the knees. Ladies, by spreading your knees apart as far as possible, you can increase the depth of penetration for your partner.

Take advantage of this face-to-face position by making eye contact, talking, and kissing. And who can resist a little nibble to the neck and ears? Guys, this is a face-to-breast position too! You've got your hands, tongue, and mouth. Drive her wild with them! Even though your legs are pinned down, you can still help with the thrusting. As you approach orgasm, grip her buttocks to help move her up and down. This could be the best taxi ride of your lifetime!

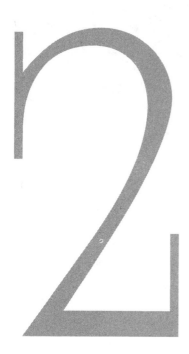

MONTH 2

Day 1. Touch Your Toes

Day 2. Blowing Hot and Cold

Day 3. Great Balls of Fire

Day 4. Hanging Out in the

　　　　Hammock

Day 5. Kneeling for the Queen

Day 6. A Shoulder to Lean On

Day 7. Chest Press

Day 8. Blind Man's Bluff

Day 9. In Seventh Heaven

Day 10. Let Your Fingers

　　　　Do the Talking

Day 11. Love Me Tender

Day 12. Up, Down, and Sideways

Day 13. Blow Your Brains Out

Day 14. Not Your Parents'

　　　　Missionary

Day 15. Busy as a Bee

Day 16. Two in Hand,

　　　　One in the Bush

Day 17. Is This Seat Taken?

Day 18. Bottoms Up!

Day 19. Play the Hand You're Dealt

Day 20. Keep Your Pecker Up

Day 21. The Electrical Chair

Day 22. Batteries Required

Day 23. In a New York Minute

Day 24. Lick into Shape

Day 25. Banana Splits

Day 26. Dangerous Intersection

Day 27. Tying the Knot

Day 28. Screwdriver

Day 29. May Cause Swelling

Day 30. Back Seat Driver

Touch Your Toes

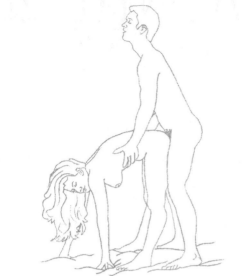

Sizzling —

Hot —

Warm —

Cold —

Calisthenics and sex at the same time? Well, not exactly! This position is great because it's both a rear-entry and a standing position.

Ladies, you need to bend down and put your hands on the floor. True toe touches require your legs to be straight and your feet to be together. But for this toe touch, spread your feet apart and bend your legs slightly at the knees. Rest your weight on your hands and get comfortable.

Guys, you'll be doing the thrusting on this one. Stand behind your partner and bend your knees as necessary to attain the correct height for penetration. If your partner is a lot shorter than you, she may need to stand on something to make her taller. Maneuver your partner's hips to help guide your penis into her vagina. Once in, keep your hands on her buttocks and hips to help her maintain her balance, and thrust away!

Blowing Hot and Cold

Month 2
Day 2

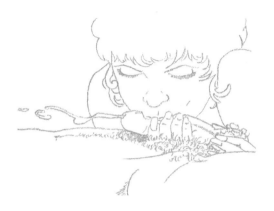

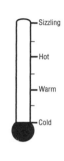

Her wet tongue. Her hot breath. A cold chill?

This is a very intense fellatio activity!

Ladies, pick a fellatio position that you like and get comfortable. Lick a small spot on the shaft of the man's penis and then blow air on it. The feel of the air hitting the wet skin produces an intense chill that will send a shiver up the man's spine! Continue making small wet spots on the shaft of his penis and blowing on them. Gradually increase the size of the spots until you're licking and blowing on one entire side of his penis. Then, when he thinks it can't get any better, move to the penis head. Lick around the head of his penis and blow air onto it. With his nerves already on edge, he'll feel this all the way to his toes!

Lick and blow air onto the entire penis head one more time. Then, before the chill has a chance to wear off, take the entire penis into your hot mouth. The heat will overwhelm him! Continue using your mouth and tongue to bring him to orgasm. Chances are, he won't blow hot and cold about this activity!

Great Balls of Fire

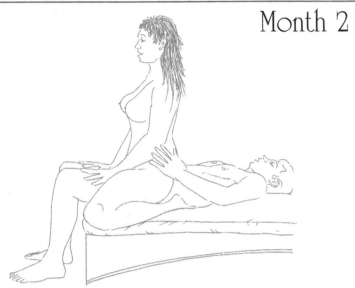

Sizzling —

Hot —

Warm —

Cold —

Lie on your back, guys, with your legs hanging over the edge of the bed. If you looked at the picture and thought, "woman on top, no need for me to do the work on this one," then you thought wrong. The reason your legs are over the side of the bed is so that your feet can reach the floor and you can use your legs to help with the thrusting.

Ladies, have the fire extinguisher ready because in this position, you get to turn up the heat by massaging your man's testicles! Sit on top, facing the man's feet with your legs by the man's hips. Your legs should be completely bent at the knees.

Reach down between the man's legs and gently grab his testicles. Rub them around between your fingers while massaging them. Lightly squeeze them, keeping tempo with his thrusting. You'll be able to tell by his reaction which techniques he likes best. This is also a great position for masturbating. But you need to start pretty early because with you setting his balls on fire, your man won't last long!

Hanging Out in the Hammock

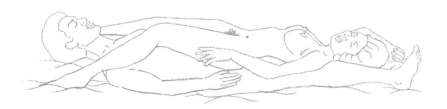

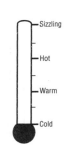

Sizzling

Hot

Warm

Cold

A lazy afternoon, a secluded hammock, and an irresistible urge. And now, a great position for swinging in the hammock! If your hammock is out in the open and you feel a little daring, stay dressed. A pair of loose track shorts for the man and a skirt for the woman, and it looks like two people taking an afternoon nap! Of course, this position works well in the bedroom too.

The man lies down on his back with his legs together.

Ladies, you get to do the rest of the work needed to get into this position. The easiest way to do this is to start by sitting on your man with your legs straight in front of you resting on his shoulders. As you sit down, use your hand to guide his penis into your vagina. Because your legs are together, the penis should have a nice snug fit! Then, with your hands next to you for support, lower yourself down until you are resting

on the man's legs.

The skin-to-skin contact with this position is wonderful! Both of you can use your hands to rub the other person's legs and hips. Ladies, if you need some clitoral stimulation, feel free to use one hand for masturbation. Neither of you has much leverage for strong thrusting. So, work together, moving your hips simultaneously to develop a smooth rhythm.

Kneeling for the Queen

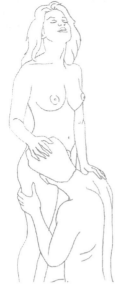

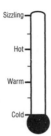

Sizzling

Hot

Warm

Cold

This expression comes from England and is used when someone is being knighted. The man becoming a knight must get down on his knees before the queen. The queen taps him on both shoulders with a sword and bestows the knighthood.

Ladies, tonight you're the queen and your partner must prove himself worthy of being a knight. Stand with your legs spread apart. This will help give the knight a better angle and also keeps you a bit more balanced.

You'll be thankful for this as you approach orgasm!

Okay guys, on your knees! Your goal is to stimulate your partner to the point where standing on two feet becomes a challenge. Using one hand to help hold her steady, start kissing the top of her thighs. These kisses should be very light and ticklish. Slowly, start moving the kisses over to her labia, using your tongue to move the folds of skin back and forth. Circle the area around her clitoris with your

tongue, making the circle smaller and smaller each time. Finally, put your entire mouth around her clitoris. This very intense action will be enough to cause an instantaneous orgasm for many women! If it does, keep going, because she'll probably have more. With your mouth still surrounding her clitoris, rub your tongue back and forth until she orgasms. Then, for the rest of the night, insist on being called Sir since your knighthood is now official!

A Shoulder to Lean On

Month 2
Day 6

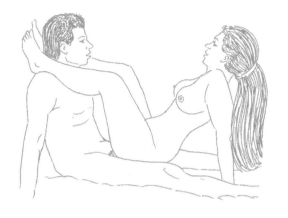

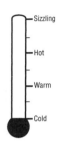

The angle of the woman makes this a very deep and satisfying position!

The man sits on the bed with his legs spread open wide. Ladies, facing your man, start by lowering yourself onto his penis. Let him use his hands to guide your hips to the right spot so that you can smoothly slide down the shaft. To make the penetration even deeper, lean backward with your arms straight behind you. This will significantly open up the walls of the vagina. Then, lift your legs so they are resting on the man's shoulders. Squeeze them together to give him a little leg hug!

Either or both of you can do the thrusting on this one. With your legs spread open, guys, it's a little harder to get leverage. But if you grasp the woman's hips with your hands and push them down while you thrust your hips up, you'll have no difficulty generating enough friction to orgasm! Ladies, you can definitely help out here. Your weight should be resting on your arms. So, move your hips forward and backward to take you up and down the shaft of the penis. Many of you will be pleasantly surprised to find out that this position can cause intense G-spot stimulation!

Chest Press

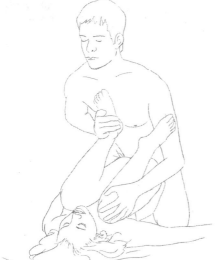

Sizzling
Hot
Warm
Cold

Guys who want to develop their pectoral muscles should do chest presses at the gym. Guys looking for a fun intercourse position should do the chest press described here!

The woman lies on her back with her legs bent up to her chest. A pillow or two will be needed under her hips to elevate them to a height where the man can insert his penis. The man kneels down and leans forward, guiding his penis inside his partner. Once inside, his hands are placed on the bed so that his arms can support most of his weight. As he leans over her, the woman should press her feet up into the man's chest.

Ladies, the closer your legs are to your chest, the deeper the man can penetrate. Tease him a bit. Straighten your legs enough so that he can maintain only a very shallow penetration. Then bend your legs completely back to your chest allowing him to fully experience the moist warmth of your vagina. Alternate between straightening your legs and bending them until he starts approaching orgasm. Then, let him maintain deep penetration for a fully satisfying climax.

Blind Man's Bluff

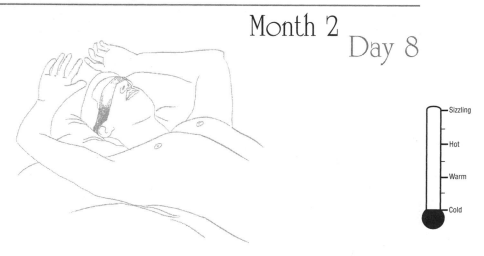

Sizzling

Hot

Warm

Cold

Ladies, start this activity by blindfolding your partner. Use something soft and silky, making sure that it's tied tight enough that he can't peek! Tell him to lie back and enjoy!

The best part of this activity is that the man has no clue what you'll be doing! It is human nature that when we see things, such as a hand getting near our leg, we anticipate what it will feel like. This brain activity diminishes the sensory stimulation. A hand touching our skin unexpectedly draws a much stronger physical response than if we can see the hand ahead of time. So, randomly touching a variety of body parts will be the key to an intensely physical experience for your partner.

This activity always ends with manual stimulation of the man's penis. However, how each of us gets to that point is extremely diverse. Focus on a variety of body parts — feet, legs, stomach, chest, arms, and neck. Use many different touching styles to tickle, massage, pinch, caress, stroke, or lightly slap. Randomly select areas of the body. For example, after massaging his feet, move to his chest rather than to his legs.

Eventually, grasp the shaft of his penis with your hand and firmly stroke him several times. If he's not peeking from under his blindfold, this will be an intensely pleasurable shock to his system! If he can stand it, go back to massaging another body part and then come back to the penis again. Finally, use your hand to manually stimulate the head and shaft until your partner orgasms.

In Seventh Heaven

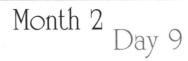

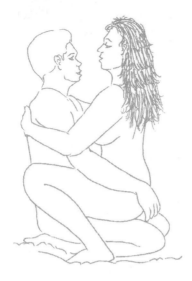

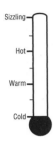

Sizzling

Hot

Warm

Cold

The man kneeling in this position will experience a bit of heaven here on earth!

Guys, you need to kneel with your legs completely underneath you so that your butt is resting on your heels. Ideally, your thighs will be flat, giving your partner a convenient spot to sit. If you can't get your buttocks all the way to your feet, your thighs will be at a downward angle from hip to knee. This is okay, as long as you keep your hands on your partner's bottom to keep her from slipping!

Ladies, straddle the man's lap facing him and lower yourself directly onto his penis. Use your hand to hold his penis upright as you slide down the shaft. Bend your legs so that your feet are flat on the floor next to the man's hips.

The benefits of this position hardly need to be pointed out! Both of you have two free hands. Use them to stroke, caress, and massage your partner. Guys, put a hand behind the woman's neck, lower her face to yours, and engage her in a deep sensuous kiss. Whisper to each other. This is a great chance to let your partner know how sexy they are and how much you love them!

Let Your Fingers Do the Talking
Month 2
Day 10

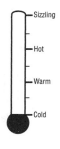

Sizzling

Hot

Warm

Cold

Actions speak louder than words. So, guys, on this one, your fingers will be saying it all!

The woman lies on her back with her legs over the edge of the bed. Spread your legs apart wide so the man has plenty of room.

Guys, kneel down between the woman's legs and start the conversation by lightly stroking her inner thighs, going from the top of the thigh down to her knees. Slide your hand back to the top of her leg and softly tickle her inner thigh. Move your fingers over and gently massage the areas around her vagina. Insert a finger or two into her vagina. When you feel the wetness of her arousal you'll know your fingers are definitely speaking her language. Leisurely work your finger up to her clitoris, spreading her labia apart as you go. With a couple of fingers, use a circular motion to massage around her clitoris. Finally, when you think your fingers have said enough, rub back and forth directly over the clitoris to bring her to orgasm. Your fingers might be talking, but your partner will be screaming!

Love Me Tender

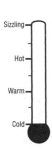

Sizzling

Hot

Warm

Cold

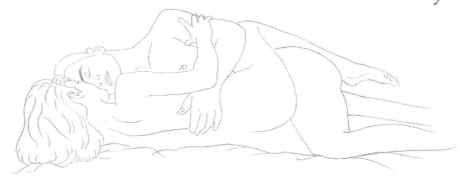

This romantic side-by-side position is perfect for cuddling, kissing, and expressing love.

Personally, I had always found side-by-side positions to be a bit tricky to accomplish. Body parts just weren't in the right spots for good penetration. But then, I learned the secret. You don't start out side to side; you move to that position after penetration has already occurred!

So, start by getting into the standard man-on-top missionary position. Then, carefully, roll together onto your sides. You should be doing most of the work here, guys. You should start moving to your side first, making sure your partner stays close and rolls with you. Ladies, once you're on your side, take your leg and drape it around the man's waist for a little extra closeness.

The biggest benefit of lying side to side is that neither of you needs to use your hands to support your weight. Your faces are right next to each other and your hands are free to caress and explore. Talk quietly, telling your partner about his or her most lovable qualities. This position is like a warm hug, but with a special bonus at the end!

Up, Down, and Sideways

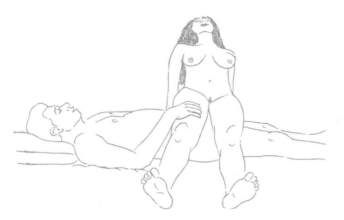

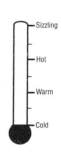

This is a very tight position with a wonderfully unique angle of penetration!

The man lies on his back with his legs out straight in front of him. The woman is on top, but rather than face the man's head or feet, she gets to sit sideways. Although similar to the Sidesaddle position used in Month 1, straightening the woman's legs and having her lean backward makes this position feel completely new.

Ladies, facing sideways, lower yourself down onto the man's penis. For maximum tightness, extend your legs straight in front of you and keep them as close together as possible. Then, lean backward using your arms to support your weight. Thrust your hips forward and backward, up and down, and from side to side. Vary the direction, pace, and depth of the thrusts to keep the man guessing what kind of sensation he'll be feeling next!

The unusual sideways penetration, the tightness of the legs, plus the angle of the vagina from the woman leaning backward, combine to produce a powerfully orgasmic experience!

Blow Your Brains Out

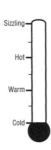

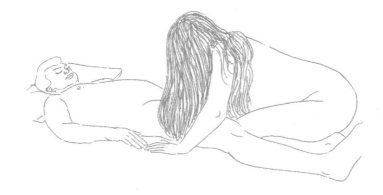

Guys, you have an easy job for this one. Lie on your back with your legs spread wide open. Now, all you have to do is enjoy!

Ladies, this fellatio position has you blowing the only brain he has working at the moment! Kneel down between the man's legs. He knows this is a fellatio position and is eager for you to get started, but don't feel inclined to rush. Start by putting your hand around his testicles and giving them a gentle squeeze. Put your other hand at the base of his penis.

Using your tongue, make long strokes up and down the shaft of his penis, avoiding any contact with the ultra-sensitive penis head. While you're doing this, remember to continue using your hands to massage his testicles and hold the base of his penis.

When you're ready, and you think your partner is more than ready, lean over and put the head of his penis into your mouth. So hot! So wet! Move your mouth up and down the shaft, mimicking vaginal penetration. For a little extra friction, use the hand from the base of the penis to move up and down the shaft simultaneously with your mouth. He'll be blowing his brains out in no time!

Not Your Parents' Missionary

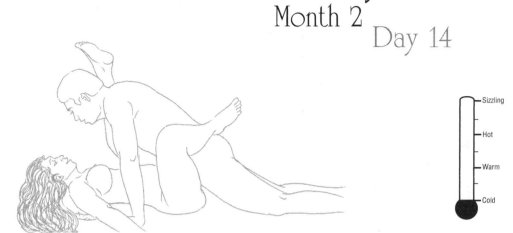

Sizzling

Hot

Warm

Cold

Tonight we have a missionary position with an interesting twist. The woman lies on her back, just like in the standard missionary position, but has one leg around the man's waist and one leg resting on the man's shoulder. Such subtle changes to the position of the woman's legs cause significant changes to the angle of the vagina and the depth of penetration!

Ladies, this is a wonderful opportunity to flex some muscles, specifically, your vaginal muscles. After the man has achieved penetration and has been thrusting a few times, constrict your vaginal muscles and hold them tight. The next time he thrusts, the extra friction will feel like a soft hand grabbing hold of his penis. Let him experience this for a few thrusts, and then relax your muscles. He'll feel your vagina loosen up. Continue alternating between flexing and relaxing. Keep him guessing what each thrust will feel like by varying the amount of time you spend doing each. Don't be surprised if he doesn't last long with this position!

Busy as a Bee

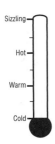

Sizzling
Hot
Warm
Cold

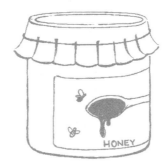

HONEY

Guys, you get to play with your food, specifically sweet, sticky honey!

For this cunnilingus activity, we start at the top and work our way down. So, get your honey and your bottle of honey and get started. Begin by putting small dots of honey from her neck all the way to the top of her breasts. Slowly and seductively lick each spot clean. Drizzle honey onto her breasts, licking all around to make them nice and wet. Use your fingers to rub the honey into her nipples before sucking it off. Sprinkle drops of honey from her breasts down her tummy to the top of her pubic hair. Fill her navel and use your tongue to lick it out. Finally, drip honey onto her genitals. It's time to stimulate her hot, sweet, sticky clitoris. Use your tongue to lick up the honey, rubbing it round and round on her clitoris. If you want, you can drip additional honey onto her genitals each time you've licked her clitoris clean. Increase your tongue's pace and pressure until your partner orgasms.

Two in Hand, One in the Bush

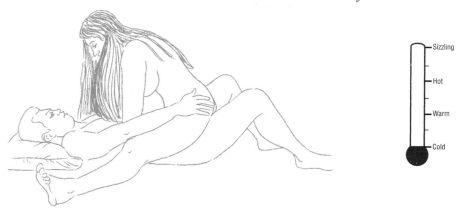

Sizzling

Hot

Warm

Cold

All your life, you've been told that one in the hand is better than two in the bush. And while that might be true if you're talking about birds, it certainly isn't true if you're talking about sex!

The man lies on his back with his legs bent at the knees. The woman sits on top of the man facing the man's head with her legs spread open as wide as possible. Then, the woman leans forward. Not only does this put the man and woman closer to each other, it also changes the angle of the vagina and allows deeper penetration. You've now succeeded at getting one in the bush.

Guys, it's time to get two in the hands. When your partner leans forward, her breasts come within your reach. Do the obvious thing here and stimulate them! If her nipples are not taut, rub your fingers against them until they get hard. Then, using your finger and thumb, gently roll her nipple back and forth. Give the nipple a little squeeze, but remember you're not trying to cause pain. The sharpness will send a tingle down her spine. Alternate between gentle and sharp, gentle and sharp. The sensations will drive her wild — and I have a feeling you'll enjoy it too!

Is This Seat Taken?

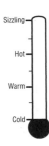

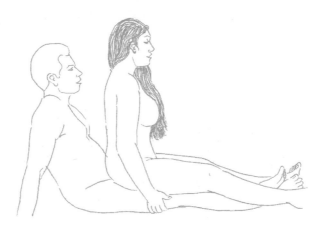

Okay, guys, here's your chance. Look her in the eyes and tell her "No sweetheart, I've been saving it for you."

The man sits with his legs straight in front of him. Ladies, you're going to sit in the man's lap facing the same direction your partner is facing. Using one hand to guide his penis, position yourself so that when you sit down, his penis slides smoothly into your vagina. Spread your legs wide open in front of you. Not only will this feel comfortable, it also gives the man direct access to your clitoris.

Guys, reach around your partner to manually stimulate her. Rub your fingers back and forth across her clitoris as she moves up and down the shaft of your penis. Increase the tempo of your fingers as she increases the tempo of the thrusting. Hold your orgasm until both of you are ready. Your partner has found the best seat in the house!

Bottoms Up!

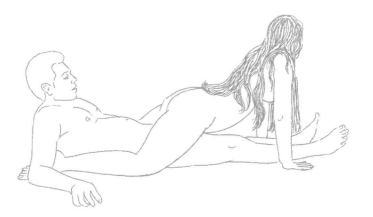

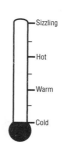

- Sizzling
- Hot
- Warm
- Cold

Finish your drinks — you've got better things to do with your hands than hold a glass!

Guys, you're on your back for this one. But instead of lying down flat, bend your arms behind you and rest your weight on your elbows. This will elevate your head and shoulders to give you a better view of your partner, especially her back and bottom!

Ladies, start this position by kneeling with your legs on either side of the man's hips. You should be facing his feet. Lower yourself onto his penis. Then, without disrupting penetration, lean forward so that your arms are straight and supporting your weight. Straighten out your legs behind you. Bump your clitoris up

against the man's pelvis each time you thrust. Not only will he find this arousing, it also provides the deepest possible penetration. Not to mention, of course, that it will also help you reach orgasm. Increase the pace of your thrusts as your orgasm develops.

Play the Hand You're Dealt

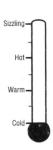

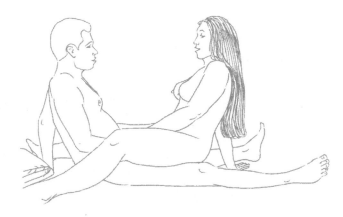

Some couples might find this position awkward because they've never masturbated in front of each other before. Give it a try. You might feel a little self-conscious at first, but stay with it. The pleasure you feel makes it all worthwhile!

This is a very intimate dual-masturbation position. The man sits with his legs straight in front of him. The woman sits on the man's thighs with her legs on either side of the man's hips. Ladies, be careful not to sit too close. Although normally maximum skin contact is encouraged, in this position, you need the extra room for your hands.

While masturbating yourself, pay attention to your partner. Guys, start by kissing your partner's neck and work your way down until you're kissing her breasts. Put your mouth around her entire areola and flick your tongue back and forth against the hard nipple. Ladies, you only need to use one hand to masturbate. Use your other hand to stroke your partner's chest and rub his nipples. Men find this very stimulating. When it looks as if your partner is approaching orgasm, increase your own tempo so that the two of you can climax at the same time.

Keep Your Pecker Up

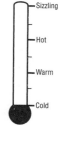

Sizzling

Hot

Warm

Cold

This is a nineteenth-century expression that means to keep your courage. Today, it means something else entirely! So, keep your pecker up for this position.

The man lies on his back with his legs straight out. Ladies, you're on top for this one, but you'll be facing the man's feet. To facilitate a velvety smooth penetration, put your mouth around the man's penis and get it nice and wet. Now you're ready to climb on. Put your feet on either side of the man's hips and lower yourself onto his penis. Bend your legs so that your knees are up by your chest. Using your feet to push off, lift your bottom up and down the shaft of his well-lubricated penis.

Guys, use your hands to help your partner with the thrusting. Put them under her buttocks to help move her up and down. This position is wonderfully deep. Keeping your pecker up should be pretty easy!

The Electrical Chair

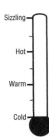

Sizzling

Hot

Warm

Cold

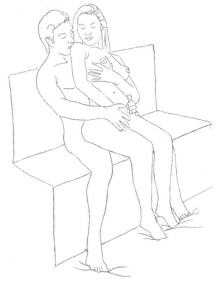

Ladies, this is a great position to use when your husband is sitting watching TV. Start by standing in front of the screen and erotically strip off your clothes. Then, walk over, sit in his lap, and grind your hips around. Once he's turned off the TV and put down the remote, stand up so he can take off his pants.

This is a great chair position that is sure to generate some electricity. The man sits comfortably in the chair and the woman sits on the man's lap facing away from the man. For really tight penetration, the woman should keep her legs close together in front of her.

Guys, with your feet on the floor, your legs should have enough leverage to do some of the thrusting. Reach your hands around to the front of your partner and lightly tickle her tummy and sides from her waist all the way to her armpits. The light sensual touch is very stimulating. Slowly move your hands to massage her breasts and nipples. For extra closeness, encourage her to lean backward against you while you're doing this. The energy will be electrifying! So, flip the switch and feel the juice!

Batteries Required

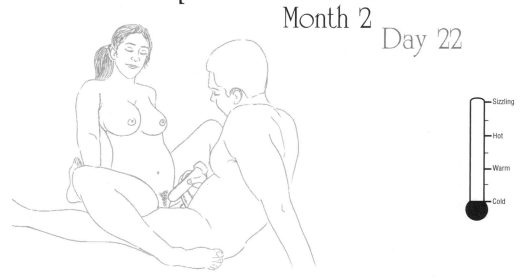

Sizzling

Hot

Warm

Cold

Make sure you have lots of spare batteries because this is the first of many vibrator activities you'll be participating in this year. Adding a vibrator to intercourse significantly increases the intensity of the orgasm.

For this activity, the man is going to use the vibrator to stimulate the woman during intercourse. This, obviously, requires a position where the man has access to the woman's clitoris while simultaneously maintaining penile penetration. Positions where the man sits or lies on his back with the woman sitting facing him are usually good for this. Make sure the woman's legs are spread open so that you get full and direct access to her clitoris. If you need help finding a suitable position, use one of the suggested positions listed below.

Once fully penetrated, start by using the vibrator to stimulate the areas around the clitoris. It's such an intense feeling that even indirect clitoral stimulation can cause many women to experience small orgasms.

Continue using the vibrator around the clitoris until you feel your own orgasm approaching. At that point, rub the vibrator back and forth directly against the woman's clitoris, bringing the two of you to a simultaneous orgasm.

Oh, and don't forget to put batteries on the grocery list!

Suggested positions: Month 1/Day 25 — Attached at the Hips; Month 3/Day 17 — Plug It In; Month 6/Day 12 — Table for Two Please; Month 8/Day 16 — Mixed Nuts; Month 11 /Day 21 — Horsing Around.

In a New York Minute

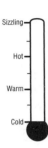

Sizzling

Hot

Warm

Cold

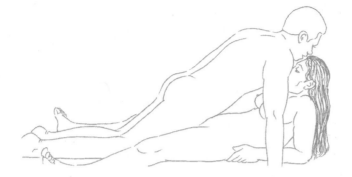

Even New Yorkers will want to take more than a minute to enjoy this position! There is no need to rush. Enjoy a nice, slow easy pace.

Ladies, the New York state motto is "excelsior." Latin for "ever upward," and this is exactly what you want your partner to be. Lower your mouth over your partner's penis and be certain that it's pointing in an upward direction. Once the state motto has been fulfilled, lie on your back with your legs open as wide as possible. Bend your arms behind you and rest your weight on your elbows.

Guys, enjoy the great geography you can find in New York. Kneel down between your partner's legs. New York has lots of rivers and waterways, so lubrication should not be an issue. As you lean toward your partner, insert your penis deep inside her warm, wet Erie Canal. Once you've fully penetrated, balance your weight on one arm while you use your other hand to massage and stimulate her Adirondack Mountains.

Use a combination of deep and shallow thrusts to increase the arousal and heighten the anticipation. Thrust your penis deep into your partner's vagina. After a few deep strokes, pull your penis nearly completely out and thrust with just the head. Thrust it in deep again several more times. And again, pull it nearly all the way out. Continue alternating this way until you approach orgasm. Once both of you are near your peaks, thrust as deep as possible until both of you have climaxed.

Now you can go enjoy some New York style pizza and cheesecake. Unless, of course, you decide you need to do this position again in a New York minute!

Lick into Shape

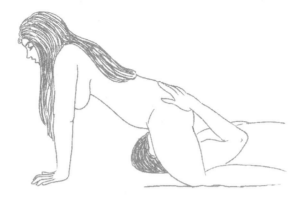

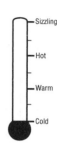

Sizzling

Hot

Warm

Cold

The man lies on his back for this cunnilingus position. Ladies, straddle the man so that your arms are above the man's head and are supporting your weight, your legs are straight behind you on either side of his hips, and, most importantly, your pelvis is directly over his face.

The rest is up to you, guys! Grasp the woman's buttocks with your hands and firmly lower her vulva to your face. Use your tongue to spread apart the labia and then insert your tongue into her vagina. Keeping your tongue pointed to provide the most pressure, dart your tongue in and out of the vagina, stimulating the nerves at the vaginal opening. Eventually, your tongue should work its way up to her clitoris. Keeping the tongue flat to cover the most surface area at a time, lick back and forth over the clitoris, increasing the pressure and speed until the woman climaxes. Enjoy the sensation as the woman grinds her hips into your face from sheer pleasure.

Banana Splits

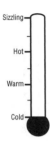

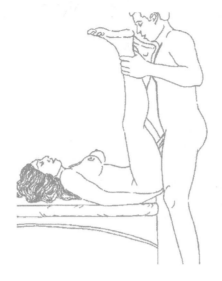

Guys, you bring the banana because the woman will be doing the splits.

The woman lies on her back with her bottom all the way forward to the edge of the bed. The guy stands next to the bed holding the woman's legs straight up into the air in front of him. Using her hands, the woman should guide the man's penis to her vagina. It might be necessary for her to put a pillow under her hips to get her to the right height for penetration.

Spread the woman's legs apart as wide as you can, guys (without making it uncomfortable for her). This gives you a very sensuous view of your penis sliding in and out of her vagina. Encourage your partner to masturbate herself. Feel her clench her vaginal muscles around your penis as she brings herself to orgasm. The sensations are enough to make you orgasm too!

Dangerous Intersection

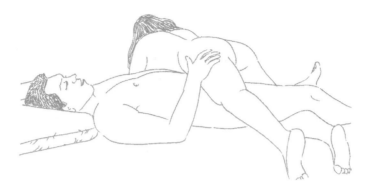

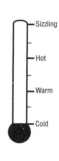

Sizzling

Hot

Warm

Cold

No stop signs at this intersection. Just full speed ahead!

Ladies, you'll be directing traffic. Have the man lie on his back with his legs straight out in front of him. Lie down on the man sideways, keeping one of your legs entwined with one of his legs. Your arms should be bent in front of you so that you can rest your weight on your elbows.

Penetration can be a little tricky in this position, so make sure the man's penis is well lubricated and that your vagina is wet. You want everything to be nice and slippery! Remember, the man's penis is pointing upward and you are pointing sideways. You need to manuever your hips around until you find an angle where he can slide right in. The other option is to start by lying down on the man with your head up by his shoulder and then rotating to the side after penetration has occurred.

Ladies, your pubic bone is resting on the man's hips. Wiggle around until you find a spot where your clitoris gets stimulated each time you thrust. Then, start your engine. You'll be driving through this intersection regularly!

Tying the Knot

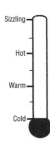

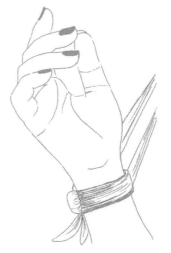

You're not getting married or renewing your vows. You're participating in a little bondage fun!

Guys, get some soft rope, nylons, or silk scarves. You can either tie the woman's hands together or tie each hand to something.

This activity requires a certain amount of trust and honesty between the couple. If the woman wants to be untied, for any reason, the man must agree that he will do this. If the situation arises, the man must keep his promise and untie the woman's hands. Women, trust your partner. This is meant to be fun!

Guys, once your partner's hands are tied, start driving her crazy with your hands. Tickle her up and down her arms. Caress her face and neck. Lightly rub her breasts and tummy. Focus on the spots you know she likes the most. If you're not sure where her favorite spots are, ask her! You might be surprised by her answer.

Ultimately, work your way to her genitals. Lightly brush your hands through her pubic hair. Run your fingers down her labia from her clitoris to her vagina and back up again. Gently massage her clitoris with your fingers, feeling its fullness as the stimulation causes it to become enlarged. Let her hips rock back and forth under your fingers until she reaches her peak.

And finally, don't forget to untie her.

Screwdriver

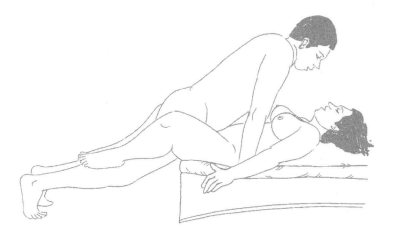

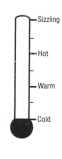

Sizzling

Hot

Warm

Cold

Get out your toolboxes, guys. You need to use your screwdriver to do a little screwing!

The woman lies on her back with her legs over the edge of the bed. The man leans against the bed with his legs out behind him and his weight resting on his arms in front of him. The man should lower his hips until they are even with the bed to ensure a straightforward and easy insertion. Once the head of the screwdriver has been inserted, start tightening!

Ladies, rest your feet on the back of the man's calves. Use your hands to tickle his sides, massage his back, and stroke the hair on his chest. Draw his head down so that he can kiss the top of your breasts. Tell him what a great maintenance man he is and how great he handles that screwdriver!

May Cause Swelling

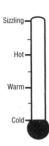

Sizzling

Hot

Warm

Cold

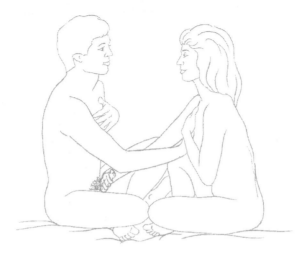

For this masturbation activity, the man and the woman are sitting facing each other. The woman should be sitting with her legs crossed underneath her. Guys, you can sit cross-legged too, or have your legs out straight and opened wide enough for the woman to sit between them. The woman needs to sit as close to the man as possible so that she can easily reach his penis with her hands.

Women, interlace your fingers and use both hands to completely encircle the man's penis. Alternate moving each of your wrists to cause a circular motion around the shaft. Gradually introduce an up-and-down motion at the same time, starting small and working up to full shaft stimulation. As the intensity increases and the man approaches orgasm, switch to one hand, firmly stroking up and down the shaft of the penis.

A few minutes after orgasm, the swelling should subside. Repeat the treatment, as needed, if the swelling returns.

Back Seat Driver

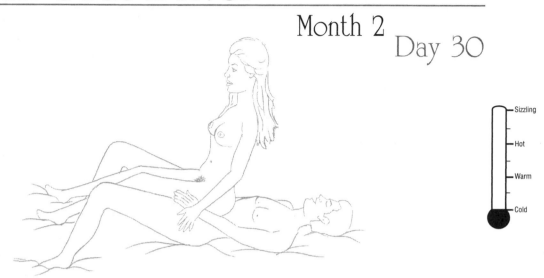

Sizzling

Hot

Warm

Cold

Men, you're on your back in this position, but with your legs bent, you can be a back seat driver.

The woman sits on the man facing the man's feet. Push your legs together as close as possible, letting your vaginal muscles give his penis a soft, tight squeeze.

Guys, this is your chance to start driving. Push off with your feet to lift and lower your hips. Put your hands on the woman's hips to keep her from moving around. Women love feeling the strong hands of their lover holding them in place during sex! Keep driving,

steadily increasing the speed, until you orgasm.

Listen, guys, I wouldn't try this in the car. Letting you be a back seat driver in the bedroom doesn't mean she'll put up with it on the street!

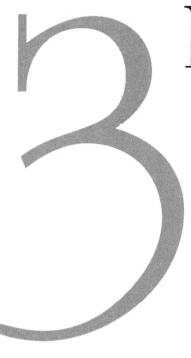

MONTH 3

Day 1. To Have and to Hold

Day 2. Sitting Down on the Job

Day 3. Head Honcho

Day 4. Man on a Mission

Day 5. Reserved Seat

Day 6. Slip Sliding Away

Day 7. Best Laid Plans

Day 8. Here Kitty, Kitty, Kitty

Day 9. Split Decision

Day 10. Keep in Touch

Day 11. Poker Player's Special

Day 12. Turn the Other Cheek

Day 13. Double Play

Day 14. Who Let the Dog Out?

Day 15. In the Hot Seat

Day 16. Sealed with a Kiss

Day 17. Plug It In

Day 18. Power Surge

Day 19. Bend Over Backward

Day 20. Side Effects

Day 21. Eating at the Y

Day 22. Manna from Heaven

Day 23. Three-Legged Race

Day 24. Side Splitting

Day 25. Early Bird Gets the Worm

Day 26. Jumping the Gun

Day 27. Dressed to Thrill

Day 28. X-tacy

Day 29. Up Your Alley

Day 30. Hands-On Training

To Have and to Hold

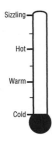

Sizzling

Hot

Warm

Cold

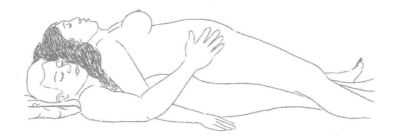

Until orgasm do you part. It's time to renew those marriage vows. This position is the perfect way to have her and hold her!

The man lies on his back with his legs out straight in front of him. The woman starts by sitting on top of the man facing the man's feet. Her legs should be spread wide open. After establishing penetration, the woman leans backward all the way to the man's chest.

Ladies, there are not a lot of places to put your hands on this one, so masturbation is definitely your best option. Move your hips up and down on the man's penis while rubbing your clitoris with your hand. You control the pace on this one, so speed up and slow down to suit your needs.

Guys, put your arms around your partner and give her a tight squeeze. Blow on her neck. Nibble on her ear. Put your hands on her breasts and massage them. Remind your partner that having her and holding her are still important to you!

Sitting Down on the Job

Month 3
Day 2

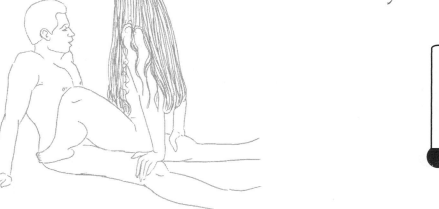

Sizzling

Hot

Warm

Cold

Sitting down is the only way to get this job done! And, what a terrific job it is!

The man sits with his legs spread open in front of him. Ladies, you will be sitting on the man's lap facing him. Straddle your partner, bending your legs so that you have a foot by each of his hips. Move your hips as close to the man's torso as possible to get the deepest, most stimulating penetration.

Run your fingers through his hair. Guys love to feel their scalp tingle! Pull his head forward and smother his face with your breasts.

Introduce a little variety to the thrusting by moving your hips from side to side, in addition to moving them up and down.

Check the job description on this one because work has never been as fun as this!

Head Honcho

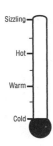

Sizzling

Hot

Warm

Cold

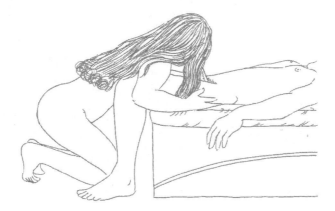

He might think he's the head honcho, but, ladies, we know the truth! And, after this fellatio position, he'll know the truth too!

The man lies on his back with his legs bent over the edge of the bed. Ladies, spread his legs apart far enough so that you can kneel down between them.

Start by licking and sucking his testicles. They're not as sensitive as his penis, but he'll find it highly erotic to feel his testicles in your warm, moist mouth.

Move onward to the shaft of his penis. Point your tongue and lightly run it from the base of his penis all the way up the shaft, stopping short of the penis head. Continue doing this with your tongue, only touching your partner as you move from the bottom of his penis to the top. It feels like half a stroke and makes him desperate for more!

Finally, encircle your mouth completely around the head of his penis. The sudden heat of your mouth will send a shock through his whole body! Use your hand to manually stroke the shaft of his penis while keeping the head of the penis in your mouth. It won't take long for him to figure out who really is the head honcho.

Man on a Mission

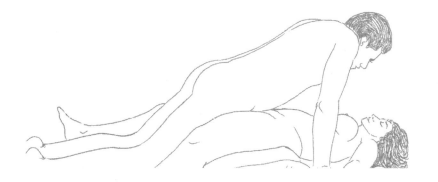

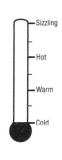

This is a missionary position where a slight change in posture produces a significant change in the overall sensations. You'll find that elevating the woman's hips greatly increases the depth of penetration.

Ladies, lie on your back with your legs spread open comfortably in front of you. Place a pillow or two under your hips to elevate them.

Guys, you'll be on top for this one. Start by kneeling between your partner's legs. Insert your finger into her vagina and use the wetness to lubricate the entire vaginal area and labia. Not only does this make her skin extra smooth, it's also highly stimulating for her! Insert your finger again and rub some of the wetness onto the head of your penis. This mission is ready for blastoff! Lean forward, inserting your penis into your partner's vagina as you stretch your legs out behind you. Enjoy the deep level of penetration you get with this position. Continue thrusting until your mission is accomplished.

Reserved Seat

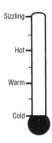

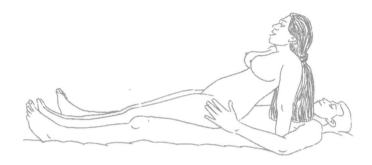

No general admission for this event! The best seat in the house has been reserved for you. And it's a hot ticket!

Guys, lie on your back with your legs spread wide open. Use your hands to grasp your partner's hips as she lowers herself onto your penis.

Ladies, you're facing the man's feet for this position.

Using your hand, insert the tip of his penis into your vagina. Lower your hips until he's penetrated about halfway and then stop. Raise your hips back up, being careful to maintain at least some penetration. Lower them again about halfway. Doing this a few times will tantalize him — he wants the nice snug feeling of full penetration!

Let him have it by lowering your hips all the way down and letting him slide completely inside of you. Put your legs straight in front of you for the tightest fit. Lean backward with your weight resting on your arms to make it the deepest fit.

Seating for this event is sure to sell out every time!

Slip Sliding Away

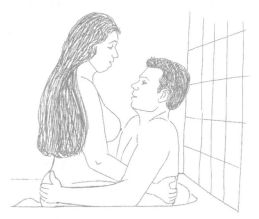

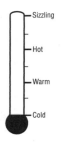

Sizzling

Hot

Warm

Cold

Water and sex make such a great combination! Wet skin is so slippery. Body parts slide back and forth so easily!

This intercourse activity is to have sex in the water. This can be done in a pool, a hot tub, or a shower, but personally, I think the bathtub works best. Fill the tub with warm, bubbly water. Light some candles and turn out the lights. Strip off your clothes, climb in, and have fun!

Start by getting each other completely wet. Use your hands and a washcloth to pour water down your partner's back, shoulders, arms, and chest. Grab the soap and take turns lathering each other up, staying away from the genitals at this point. Wash your partner's feet and suck on their toes. Cover their legs with bubbles, letting your fingers linger near the top of the thigh. Use the soap and water to make the skin silky and smooth for a wonderful back, neck, and shoulder rub. Facing your partner, get your hands extra soapy to massage their chest. Guys, rub your hands all over your partner's breasts. Squeeze them together, darting your tongue back and forth between the nipples. They feel so soft when they're wet!

Decide who gets to be on the bottom for intercourse. This person has most of their skin submerged in the warm water. It's extremely relaxing and sensual. No need for lubrication when having intercourse in the bathtub! The man's wet penis slides very easily into the woman's wet vagina. Alternate who gets to be on top or try a side-to-side position, kissing, cuddling, and thrusting until both of you have climaxed.

Afterward, dry each other off with the towels. Don't be surprised if you end up having sex again on the bathmat!

Best Laid Plans

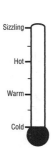

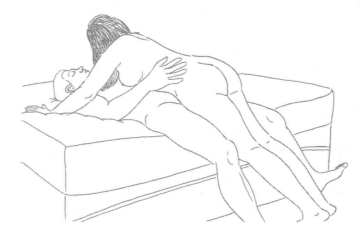

This position gives you the best laid plan to get you laid the best way!

Guys, lie on your back with your legs hanging over the edge of the bed. Your legs should be spread wide open. Ladies, you will be lying down on the man's chest with your legs out straight behind you and between the man's legs. Keep your legs together for really tight penetration. Your breasts should be pushed up against the man's chest.

This is a wonderful position for making eye contact, talking quietly, and kissing. Arouse her interest with some gentle kisses. Gradually increase the intensity until you're engaged in passionate tongue-twisting kissing!

Make plans to repeat this one again and again!

Here Kitty, Kitty, Kitty

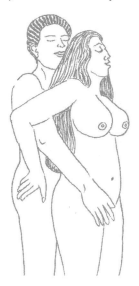

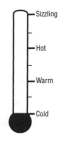

A lost pussycat in need of some petting and you're the man for the job! This is a standing position where the man manually stimulates the woman.

Ladies, stand in front of your partner, facing the same direction he's facing. Spread your legs apart.

Guys, time to go look for the kitty. This position can be a little tricky because you're standing behind the woman. You can't see what you're doing, so you'll need to rely on your sense of touch.

The easiest way to accomplish this position is to put your hand between the woman's legs from behind. Spread the labia open with your fingers as your hand moves toward the clitoral area. Feel the warmth her body is generating on your hand. As you start to stimulate the area around her clitoris, feel her hips grind into your fingers as she tries to find a spot where she can get direct clitoral stimulation. Don't give in immediately. Tease her with some indirect stimulation before rubbing your fingers directly on her clitoris. Use your other hand to keep her hips pressed up against you as she climaxes.

You'll hear this pussycat purring away!

Split Decision

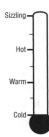

Sizzling

Hot

Warm

Cold

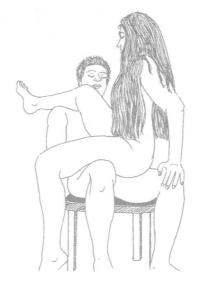

Guys, find a comfortable seat for this month's chair position!

Ladies, your seat will be on your partner's lap. Facing sideways, maneuver your hips until they are directly over the man's penis. Sit down on the man's lap, allowing him to push his penis deep into your vagina. Split your legs so that one foot is on the floor and one foot is up by your partner's neck. Not only does this allow penetration all the way to the base of his penis, it also provides an opportunity for your partner to watch you masturbate.

Remember, men are very visually stimulated, so let your fingers give him a show to watch. The combination of watching you masturbate plus feeling your vaginal muscles respond around his penis is overwhelming! Not to mention how good this will feel for you too.

No split decision here. Both of you can love this position!

Keep in Touch

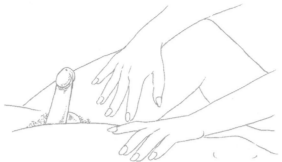

Sizzling

Hot

Warm

Cold

Relax. Breathe deep. Lie back and enjoy a massage that starts with your feet and ends with an orgasm!

Ladies, your goal with this activity is to relax all of your partner's muscles, except one. We'll focus on that muscle in a little while! Start with his feet. Hold one foot between both hands with your fingers on the bottom of the foot and your thumbs on the top. Work the thumbs and fingers together to apply pressure to the entire surface of the foot. Individually rub each toe. When you've finished one foot, move one hand then the other hand to the second foot, being careful to always maintain body contact with at least one hand.

Flatten your hands out for maximum skin contact and stroke them up and down his calves. Use your fingers and thumbs to gently knead the large muscles in the back. Delicately rub the tips of your fingers along the backs of his knees. Your fingers should barely brush his skin. Again, flatten out your hands to massage the thighs. Glide your hands up and down the thighs using more pressure as your hands move up and less pressure as your hands move down. Put your fingers together and rub small circles at the top of the inner thigh. Steadily increase the size of the circles, getting closer and closer to his perineum, testicles, and the base of his penis.

Holding his testicles in one hand, curl your other hand around the shaft of the penis and start stroking. Use your mouth to get the penis slippery and wet. This makes the stroking much smoother. Lengthen the strokes to include the very base of the penis all the way to the tip of the head. As your partner approaches his climax, use shorter and faster strokes that focus primarily on the penis head, and bring him to orgasm.

With this activity, he'll let you keep in touch as often as you want!

Poker Player's Special

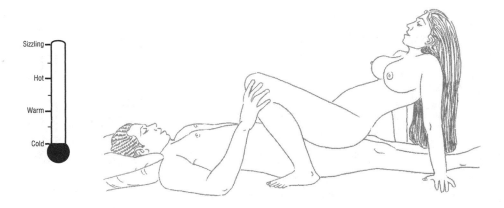

Sizzling

Hot

Warm

Cold

Guys, you'll have what every poker player wants. A partner with a great pair and your own ace in the hole!

The man lies on his back with his legs out straight. The woman sits on top of the man facing the man's head. Her legs should be completely bent so that her feet are next to the man's hips. Once penetration has occurred, the woman leans backward putting her weight on her arms. Ladies, be sure to lean backward slowly. You'll be pulling the man's penis in a direction contrary to the way it hangs naturally. When done correctly, leaning backward provides a tight fit with lots of friction and a chance for your partner to watch his penis sliding in and out of you. When not done properly . . . Well, let's just say that nobody is a winner!

Guys, no need to bluff because you've definitely got a winning hand! Use it to manually stimulate the woman's clitoris while watching her hips move up and down the shaft of your penis. Try to time the tempo of your fingers so that you both climax at the same time. She'll thank you for dealing her a royal flush!

Turn the Other Cheek

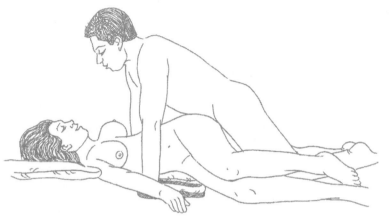

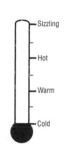

Sizzling

Hot

Warm

Cold

For this sideways penetration position, ladies, you will be lying on just one cheek. So, pick which cheek you want to turn. Then, lie on your back and twist your waist so that both of your legs are pointing to the same side. Use a pillow or two to elevate your hips.

This makes penetration much smoother!

Guys, you will be kneeling for this position. Get on your knees, leaning forward with your weight on your arms. Adjust the height of your hips so that the head of your penis lines up directly with the woman's

vagina. Have your partner help insert the penis tip and then thrust your hips forward, sinking the entire penis shaft into her soft, hot vagina. Continue thrusting using long, deep, satisfying strokes.

To do this position again, just turn the other cheek!

Double Play

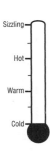

Sizzling

Hot

Warm

Cold

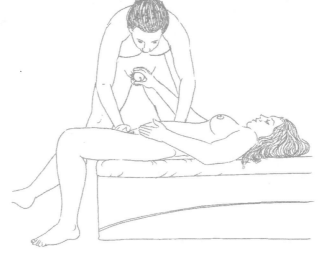

This is a nonintercourse position where each of you manually stimulates the other person.

The woman lies on her back along the edge of the bed. The man stands next to the bed by the woman's hips. He bends over to reach between the woman's legs with his hand. The woman extends her arm to grasp the man's penis with her hand.

Rather than stimulate each other simultaneously, take turns bringing each other to orgasm. It allows each of you to focus exclusively on either giving or receiving pleasure. Although typically the man will stimulate the woman first, each couple should decide the order that is right for them.

When giving pleasure, watch and read your lover's body language. Your goal is to find the spots and techniques that get the most favorable response. When receiving pleasure, be sure to let your lover know what you like best, especially when they try something new. Shift your hips, guide your lover's hand, moan, or use words. The more you communicate with your lover, the better and more satisfying your sex lives will be.

Who Let the Dog Out?

Month 3
Day 14

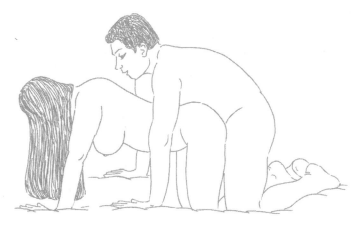

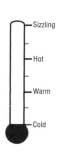

- Sizzling
- Hot
- Warm
- Cold

Doggy-style positions. You've got to love them!

Not much of a description needed for this category of positions because the name says it all. The man and woman are both on their hands and knees. The man, the top dog, penetrates the woman from behind. For this specific doggy-style position, both people have their arms straight, and the man's legs are outside the woman's legs.

Guys, kiss your lover's neck. Move her hair aside and kiss her right on the hairline. Lightly tickle her neck with your tongue. The neck is an erogenous zone for many women. Make her nerves stand on end.

Support yourself on one hand and use your other hand to manually stimulate the woman. Start with her breast and slowly move your fingers down to her clitoris, stroking, tickling, and massaging as you move along. Rub your fingers back and forth over her clitoris while you thrust your penis deep inside of her. Feel free to let your canine instincts loose and let out a howl.

In the Hot Seat

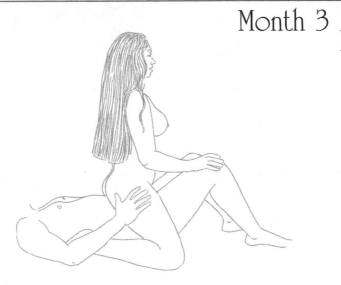

Sizzling—
Hot—
Warm—
Cold—

This one is a scorcher!

The man lies on his back with his knees bent. The woman sits on the man facing the man's feet. Her legs are bent so that her feet are behind her. Ladies, for the deepest penetration, spread your knees apart as far as you can.

The man, the woman, or both can do the thrusting for this position. Because his legs are bent, the man has enough leverage to move his hips up and down. If the woman synchronizes when she raises and lowers her hips, the full length of the man's penis will be moving in and out of her vagina. When the man lifts his hips up, the woman should lower her hips down for the deepest penetration. Conversely, when the man lowers his hips, the woman should raise hers so that nearly the entire penis shaft is removed from the vagina. Each time the penis is thrust back into the vagina, the man experiences a rush of heat as it rubs against the hot vaginal walls and generates friction.

Watch him sweat! The hot seat has never been hotter!

Sealed with a Kiss

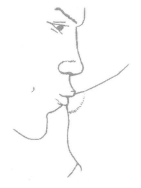

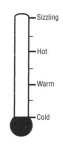

This is a cunnilingus activity that will keep your lips very busy! You will arouse and stimulate your partner by kissing her from her head down to her hips, with a final destination that is sure to be climactic.

Start by kissing her scalp while running your fingers through her hair. The tingling she feels will be just the beginning! Move down to gently kiss her forehead, eyes, and cheeks. Lightly lick her lips before pressing your lips against hers. Pretend this is the first time you've kissed your partner, and let your tongue explore her mouth.

Although it's tempting to continue the passionate kissing, continue moving on toward your final destination. Kiss her chin and neck. Drag your tongue from the tip of her chin to the base of her neck, and from the base of her neck to the top of her breasts. Holding her breast in your hand, kiss all around the breast before closing your mouth around the nipple. Let your tongue slide back and forth across it. Pull your lips back and very gently bite the nipple, holding it between your front teeth. Women find it highly erotic when they can

see and feel your teeth biting their breasts!

Give her small kisses from her breasts down her tummy to her pelvis. Bury your face in her pubic hair, kissing the skin underneath it as you move to the clitoral area. Use your tongue to spread apart her labia and explore everything from her clitoris to her vagina. Rub your tongue against her clitoris, feeling it swell. Continue rubbing your tongue back and forth until your partner orgasms.

And to think, it all started with an innocent little kiss to the scalp!

Plug It In

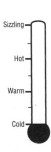

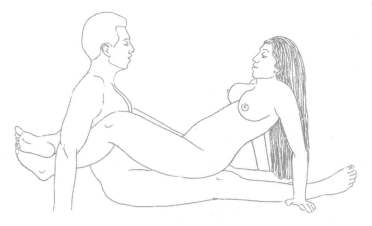

Looking for an outlet to plug in your power cord? We have just the answer!

Guys, sit on the bed with your legs straight in front of you. Be sure that your power cord is fully extended.

Ladies, you will be sitting on the man's lap with your legs wrapped around his waist. Align your hips, and then firmly grab his power cord and plug it into your socket. Lean backward onto your arms to ensure a deep, powerful connection.

Guys, while your partner is generating energy thrusting her hips, use your hand to manually stimulate her energy source. Rub your hand back and forth across her clitoris, matching the intensity and tempo of her thrusting until both of you orgasm.

System overload! Remove the power cord from the outlet and reset the circuit breakers!

Power Surge

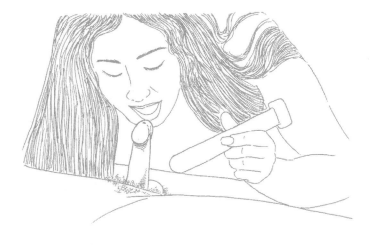

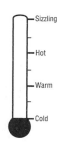

Sizzling

Hot

Warm

Cold

So, a few of you guys have never used a vibrator before? Relax! Vibrators are not just for women. Try it once and you'll be hooked.

Ladies, start by having your partner lie down and get comfortable. Let him feel the vibrator on his arms and legs. There are no words to describe that tingly feeling the vibrator produces! Move over and stroke the vibrator along his chest, letting it rest directly on the nipple for a second or two. Notice how hard his nipples get when you do this!

Run the vibrator from his chest down to the base of his penis. Slide the vibrator up and down the shaft of his penis. He'll think this is incredible, but the best is yet to come! Roll the vibrator around the head of the penis. Move it from the edge to the center, all around the edge, up the back of the head, and around the very tip. This will be almost too intense for some guys to handle!

As you slide the vibrator back down the shaft, lower your mouth onto the head

of your partner's penis. His nerves are already on edge from the vibrations. The soft heat of your mouth feels outstanding! Rub the vibrator up and down the shaft and on his testicles while the penis head moves back and forth in your mouth. Rub your tongue around the head as you move it in and out.

Warning! This activity is extremely stimulating! The power surge might be followed by a power outage!

Bend Over Backward

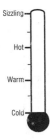

Sizzling

Hot

Warm

Cold

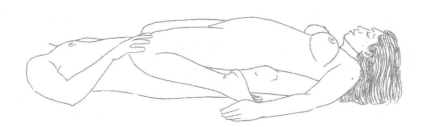

Both of you get to bend backward a little bit with this one!

The man lies on his back with his legs straight in front of him. No bending backward yet! The woman starts by sitting on the man, facing him, with one leg on each side of him. Her legs should be bent so that her feet are behind her.

Now the bending starts. Ladies, very slowly and gently lean completely backward until you are resting on the man's legs. While you are leaning backward, the man's penis will actually be bending backward. So, go slow!

Because of the angle of the penis, penetration with this position is fairly shallow. But what it lacks in depth, it makes up for with friction. It's very important to use a short thrusting stroke to prevent the penis from inadvertently being pulled out of the vagina. Unfortunately, if the penis is accidentally removed, it will return to its natural, unbent position and you'll be starting over.

Side Effects

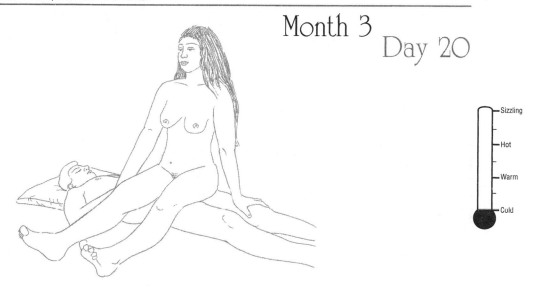

Sizzling

Hot

Warm

Cold

The side effects from this sideways position are pleasure and fun!

The man lies on his back with his legs straight in front of him. The woman sits on top of the man facing sideways. Ladies, keep your legs as close together as possible, squeezing his penis tightly inside your vagina.

Potential side effects increase with the use of hands. Ladies, reach down between the man's legs and wrap your hand around his testicles. Use your other hand to masturbate. Guys, use one hand to stroke and tickle her lower back and buttocks. Put your other hand over your partner's hand while she masturbates. Feel the position of her fingers, the firmness of her touch, and the techniques that she uses to please herself. Not only is this educational, it's also very erotic for both of you!

Eating at the Y

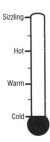

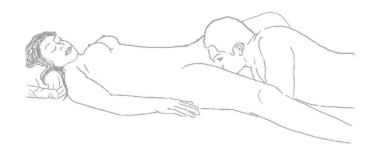

As a kid, did you ever play the game where you tried to form letters of the alphabet using your body? Maybe it was part of a cheerleading routine or a dance move. Well, ladies, for this position, you need to form the letter Y.

Guys, this is a cunnilingus position where you lie on your stomach between the woman's legs. Spread her thighs apart as far as they will go. While she's watching, seductively lick the tip of your finger and insert it into her vagina. Then lick your lips, lower your head, and put your mouth around the clitoral area. Move your finger around in a circle along the vaginal walls while moving your tongue around in a circle around the clitoris. Get her fully aroused and then pull completely back.

Sex is about more than just having an orgasm. It's also the excitement, the arousal, and the titillating events leading up to the climax. So, stimulate her.

Let her feel the pleasure and anticipation. Take her to the edge, but then temporarily delay the orgasm. Kiss and stroke her thighs, hips, and pubic hair. Occasionally, let your tongue slide across her clitoris. When the Y is ready for the big O, bring her to orgasm by putting your mouth fully around her clitoris and rubbing your tongue back and forth.

Yes! Yahoo! Yippee!

Manna from Heaven

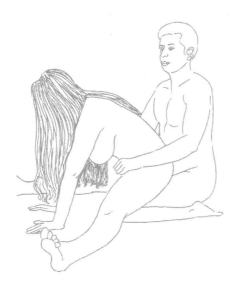

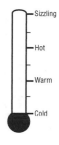

Originally, manna was the food that was miraculously provided to the Israelites in the wilderness during their exodus from Egypt. Today, manna is a windfall, an unexpected piece of good fortune, a miraculous turn of events. For the guy kneeling in this position, manna from heaven is the woman sitting on his lap!

Guys, kneel on the bed with your legs completely bent so that your bottom is resting on the back of your calves. Have your partner kneel in front of you, facing away from you, with her legs spread open wide. Reach between her legs and insert a finger into her vagina, stimulating her until she's nice and wet. Using one hand to hold your penis and the other hand to guide her hips, insert your penis into her vagina, lowering her hips down to your lap.

Ladies, keep your legs spread open as wide as you can. Lean forward and put your hands on the bed in front of you. This makes the penetration really tight, and also gives you some leverage so you can move your hips up and down the shaft of the man's penis. Each time you thrust, your partner should feel your bottom pressing into his lap. The entire length of his penis, from the tip to the base, should be surrounded by your velvety smooth and wickedly hot vagina.

Bring him to orgasm. Let him experience manna from heaven for himself!

Three-Legged Race

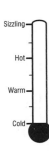

Sizzling
Hot
Warm
Cold

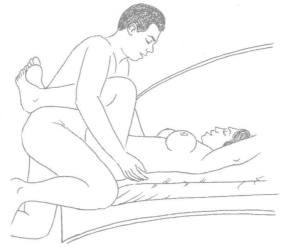

Lie on your back, ladies, with your bottom all the way to the edge of the bed. Initially, your legs will hang over the side of the bed. Wrap them around your partner's waist once he gets into position.

Guys, you provide all three legs for this race! The first leg is kneeling on the floor. The second leg is kneeling up on the bed. The third leg is ensconced deep inside the woman's vagina. Apparently, this leg thought it was a sack race.

Put most of your weight on the knee that is up on the bed. It gives you lots of leverage for thrusting and also allows your third leg to penetrate really deep. Look down and watch your penis going into and out of your partner's vagina. The visual stimulation adds a whole new level of intensity.

Manually stimulate your partner's clitoris, bringing her to orgasm while you watch her hips grind into your penis.

Everyone is a winner with this race!

Side Splitting

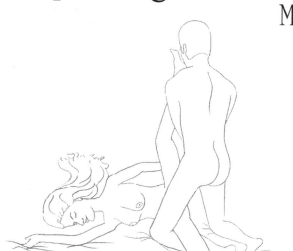

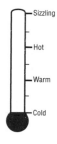

Sizzling

Hot

Warm

Cold

This position looks a bit unusual, but it's very fun! Because the woman's legs are spread so far apart, the penetration is very deep. And with the woman lying on her side, the angle of penetration is interesting and satisfying.

The woman lies on her side with a few pillows under her hips to elevate them. One leg stays on the bed and goes between the man's legs.

The other leg is extended straight into the air and rests on the man's shoulder.

Guys, kneel down next to your partner with her leg between your knees. Help her lift her other leg into the air. Her wide-spread legs give you a great view of her genitals. Spread the labia apart with your fingers and manually stimulate her clitoris. For some women, an orgasm before

intercourse increases their chances of having an orgasm during intercourse.

Position your hips so that your penis slides smoothly into her vagina. Her vagina is deep and wide from her orgasm, so thrust using the full length of your penis. Use your hands to hold her hips still while you increase the intensity of your thrusting. Clutch her to you as you reach your climax!

Early Bird Gets the Worm

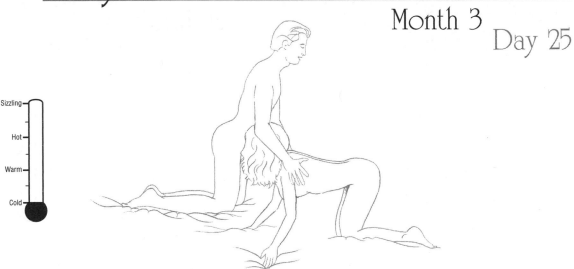

Sizzling

Hot

Warm

Cold

Ladies, get out your lip balm. This is a fellatio position, so your lips need to be nice and soft!

For this position, the man is kneeling. You will eventually be on your hands and knees, but start out by kneeling too. Rub your hands all over the man's chest. Like women, men also have sensitive nipples. Lean over and put your mouth around his entire nipple, running your tongue back and forth across the hard center.

Lower your hands so they can stroke and tickle his sides and hips. Continue leaning further down and kiss him from his chest to his belly button and then to his pubic hair. Move your hands around to his buttocks, kneading them between your fingers and thumbs. Pull him to you as you lower your head even further and put your mouth around his penis. Stroke the head of the penis with your tongue while still keeping as much of the shaft inside your mouth as possible.

Keeping your lips around his penis, move your head forward and backward allowing the penis to be thrust back and forth into your mouth as your partner begins rocking his hips. Keep things interesting by whipping your tongue around on the shaft and head while the penis is moving in and out. For increased friction, use your hand to move up and down the wet shaft simultaneously with your mouth. Increase the pace and intensity until you bring him to orgasm.

Jumping the Gun

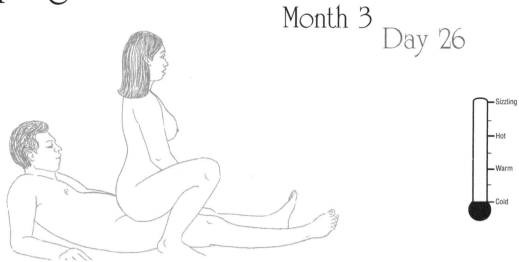

Sizzling

Hot

Warm

Cold

Although originally an expression for when runners would start a race before the gun was fired, jumping the gun in this position has nothing to do with a false start!

The man is on his back with his legs straight out in front of him. For this position, the man has his arms bent and his weight on his elbows so that he is reclining rather than lying flat.

Ladies, straddle the man, facing his feet. Your legs should be completely bent so that your feet are flat on the bed next to his hips. Poise your hips over the gun and slide the target down the gun shaft. Although the man will probably do most of the thrusting, lift and lower your hips to increase the intensity. Your legs are spread wide, so use your hand to masturbate your clitoris. No reason why you can't have some gunfire of your own!

Once your partner's chamber has been emptied into your target, put the gun away so it can be reloaded for next time. No wonder so many guys carry concealed weapons!

Dressed to Thrill

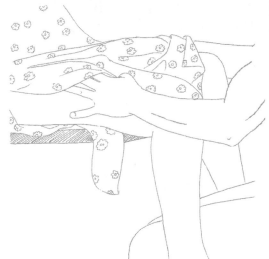

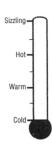

Sizzling —

Hot —

Warm —

Cold —

For this activity, the man manually stimulates his partner while she is still dressed. The beauty of this activity is that it can be done in so many places! At the movies, on an airplane, or sitting in traffic! Be creative. And be a little naughty!

How you perform this activity depends, in part, on what your partner is wearing. If she's wearing a dress or skirt, slide your hand under it and follow her thigh up to her pubic hair. If she has on panties (and you might be surprised to find out that she doesn't), move the crotch of the panties aside and get some skin-on-skin contact as you move your fingers over to her clitoris. The foot also works well under a dress and is sometimes a lot less conspicuous. Having difficulty moving the panties aside using your foot? Don't worry! Leave the panties where they are and use your big toe to massage her clitoris with her panties still in place. Silky panties feel great when they're rubbed back and forth!

If your partner is wearing pants, the trick is to use the seam of the pants to rub against the clitoris. Again, you can use either your hand or your foot. Slightly shift the seam of the pants around until you've located a sensitive spot on her clitoris. Rub the seam back and forth until the woman reaches her peak.

Oh, and when picking a place for this activity, there is one more factor to consider. Is she a screamer?

X-tacy

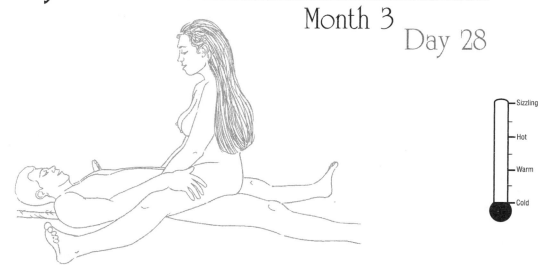

Sizzling
Hot
Warm
Cold

This x-tra special position is very x-iting and x-ilarating. With a little x-perience, you will be an x-pert in no time!

The man lies on his back with his legs spread wide open. The woman sits on top of the man, facing his head, with her legs spread wide open too.

Ladies, reach down behind you and cup your hand around your partner's testicles. Roll them around and massage the folds of skin. Use your other hand to guide your partner's hand to your clitoris. Put your fingers over his fingers and guide him to the x-act spots that you want stimulated. If you want him to rub his fingers round and round, then move his fingers round and round. If you want him to rub back and forth, then move his fingers back and forth. Together, set the intensity and the pace until both of you have reached your peak.

I think you will find this an x-tremely x-plosive x-perience!

Up Your Alley

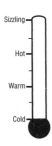

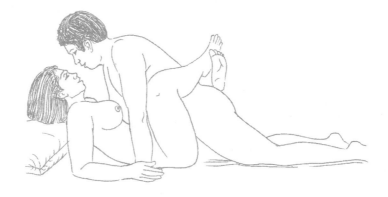

Pleasurable sex does not have to be your area of expertise for this position to be right up your alley.

The woman lies on her back, but with her weight resting on her elbows to elevate her head and shoulders. The man uses the standard missionary-type pose with his legs straight out behind him and his weight resting on his arms in front of him.

Ladies, once the man's penis has entered your vagina, lift your legs and wrap them around his waist. Squeeze his torso with your legs to bring his hips into direct contact with your clitoris. Manipulate your hips so that your alley cat gets stimulated each time your partner goes up your alley. Keep your legs wrapped tightly around your partner's waist. Guys love to be trapped by their lover's leg embrace! Let him know when you're close to peaking so that he can intensify his thrusts and climax at the same time.

Hands-On Training

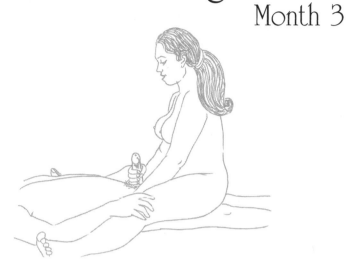

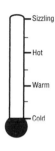

We'll finish the month with a position where the woman manually stimulates her partner.

Ladies, have your partner lie on his back with his legs out straight in front of him. Sit on the man's thighs with your pelvis up close to the man's penis.

Start the training session by rubbing the head of his penis against your inner thighs. Scoot up close enough so that you can rub his penis against your labia and clitoris. The visual stimuli he gets from watching this is very intense!

Putting one hand on each side of the shaft, rub your hands back and forth. Simultaneously, move your hands up and down the penis while rubbing the shaft between your hands. Be careful! You don't want to cause a friction burn when you do this!

Move one hand to lightly stroke the head of the penis while using the other hand to firmly stroke the shaft. Increase the length of the stroke to include the head of the penis. Enjoy feeling your partner's legs squirm as you hold him in place with your weight! The hands-on training session is complete when your partner climaxes.

Ladies, don't believe your partner when he tells you that you're not very good at this. He's just trying to get you to repeat your training!

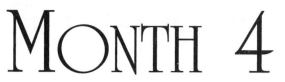

MONTH 4

Day 1. Stand By for Take-off

Day 2. The Big Picture

Day 3. Toe the Line

Day 4. Easy on the Hard-on

Day 5. Rock My World

Day 6. Make Hay While the

      Sun Shines

Day 7. Working Overtime

Day 8. A Fresh Perspective

Day 9. Blowing Your Top

Day 10. Riding Shotgun

Day 11. Chip on Your Shoulder

Day 12. Burning the Midnight Oil

Day 13. Old Friend

Day 14. The Organ Grinder

Day 15. Heads or Tails?

Day 16. All-You-Can-Eat Special

Day 17. Golfer's Delight

Day 18. Bake at 350 Degrees

Day 19. Easy Come, Easy Go!

Day 20. Blind Date

Day 21. Geometry Lesson

Day 22. Full Moon Rising

Day 23. Knee Pads Optional

Day 24. Finger Painting

Day 25. Naughty Is

      Sooooo Nice!

Day 26. Pleasant Dreams

Day 27. Take a Bow

Day 28. Diddly Squat

Day 29. Tongue-tied

Day 30. Split Personality

Stand By for Take-off

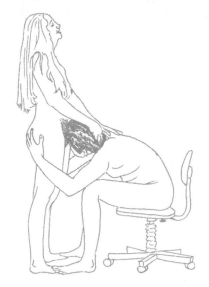

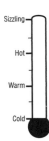

This is a cunnilingus position that will send her flying!

Guys, sit on a chair or couch with your partner standing in front of you. Check the altitude. If your partner is flying too low for you to maneuver your mouth to the right position, have her stand on a box or stool.

Firmly grasp your partner's hips and pull her to you. Spread her legs apart with your hands and rub your fingers along her clitoris as a preflight equipment check. If you feel her respond to your fingers, then the flight is ready for take-off.

Prepare for turbulence as you cover her entire clitoral area with your mouth. Keep your lips pressed firmly against her skin. You might feel the plane shaking a bit.

Use your tongue to rub back and forth against the clitoris. Make some airplane noises. The vibration of your lips is like a tiny, hot, and wet vibrator! Continue stimulating her clitoris until she has reached her final destination.

Thank you for flying. We hope you have enjoyed your flight. Please fly with us again soon!

The Big Picture

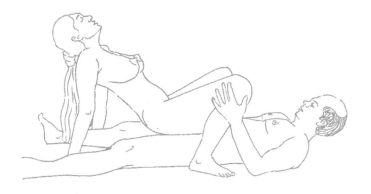

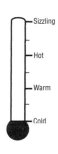

Sizzling

Hot

Warm

Cold

Don't get lost in the details. This position has definitely got the big picture!

Guys, lie on your back with your legs spread open wide. Lift your head (the one on your shoulders) so you can watch the big picture.

Ladies, you'll be sitting on your partner facing him. Your legs will be completely bent so that your feet are flat on the bed next to his hips. Start by straddling

your partner with your hips hovering over the head of his penis. Lean backward with your arms behind you to support your weight.

Lower your hips just a bit so that your lover can line up the head of his penis with your vagina. Then, very slowly, lower your hips and totally engulf your lover's penis inside of you. Your partner gets to witness a wonderfully erotic view as

the entrance to your vagina expands around his penis. Slowly raise and lower your hips, letting your partner watch as his penis slides in and out.

Support your weight on one arm and use the other hand to masturbate. Let your partner watch as you spread apart your labia. Increase the tempo of your thrusting as you and your partner both climax.

Toe the Line

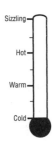

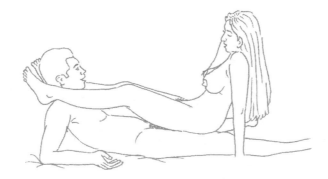

Live by the rules? Follow good behavior? Toe the line? You don't need to with this position!

The man lies on his back with his legs out straight in front of him. He bends his arms behind him so that his weight is resting on his elbows. This will elevate his shoulders and head.

The woman initiates penetration by starting out in a sitting position facing the man's head. After penetration, she places her legs on the man's chest with her feet up by his shoulders. She bends her arms and leans backward with her weight resting on her elbows.

Guys, with your partner's feet right next to your face, this is the perfect time for a little tongue and toe tango. The toes are a very sensitive erogenous zone for many people, particularly women.

Start by putting her big toe between your lips and sucking on it. No need to be particularly gentle since the skin on the toes is so thick.

Replace the big toe with all the remaining toes. Suck on them one by one. Run your tongue in the sensitive areas between them. Rub the top of her toes against your teeth while rubbing the bottom of her toes with your tongue. Have your partner wiggle her toes around while you hold them in your mouth. Making them wet and warm will make other areas wet and warm too! Thrust your hips until both of you have crossed the line.

Easy on the Hard-on

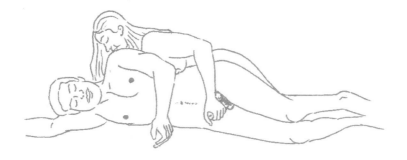

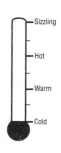

Sizzling

Hot

Warm

Cold

This is a very loving and sweet position for when the woman is manually stimulating the man. It is particularly useful first thing in the morning before getting out of bed.

The man and woman lie on their sides next to each other. Both of them are facing the same direction. For this position, the man is in front of the woman.

Ladies, reach your arm around your partner and stroke his chest and stomach. Work your way down to his groin and put your hand firmly around his penis.

Because of the physical anatomy of men and women, you rarely get to have your partner in front of you. Breathe on his neck and back. The soft blasts of warm air are very arousing for him.

Push your hips up against his buttocks for some clitoral stimulation. Draping one leg over their partner's legs offers some women a better, more satisfying angle for stimulating their clitoris. Work your hips back and forth, women, while your hand moves up and down the shaft of his penis. Your hot breath, your hips grinding into his buttocks, your hand stroking the shaft of his penis — this hard-on won't last long!

Rock My World

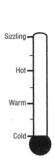

Sizzling

Hot

Warm

Cold

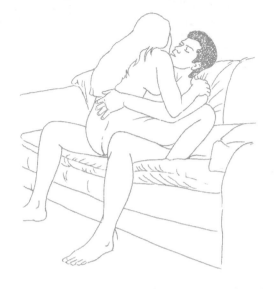

This sitting position is perfect for a rocking chair or a porch swing!

The man sits on the chair or couch with his feet on the floor. The woman sits on the man's lap facing him. Her legs are completely bent so that her feet are flat next to the man's hips.

Guys, put your arms around your partner's waist and hold her tight. If you're lucky enough to be in a rocking chair (or swing), push your feet off the floor and start rocking. The natural movement results in nearly effortless thrusting. So use your extra energy to deeply and passionately kiss your lover. Look her in the eyes and tell her how much you love her.

As your excitement builds to orgasm, lift and lower your hips to intensify the thrusting. Put your hands on your lover's buttocks to help her lift and lower her hips too. Your world will be rocking!

Make Hay While the Sun Shines

Month 4
Day 6

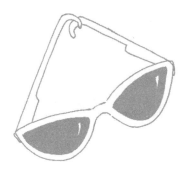

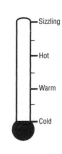

- Sizzling
- Hot
- Warm
- Cold

Sex and sunshine! Just thinking about the two subjects is almost enough to cause spring fever. If you can do this activity during the day, terrific! If not, no problem. It works at night too.

For this activity, you will have intercourse while wearing your sunglasses.

Why? Because it's light-hearted fun and a lot of people don't get enough of it. Select a position where you can see each other. If possible use mirrored sunglasses. Mirrored glasses are cool because each of you will see the reflection of things you don't ordinarily get to see.

Have fun! Laugh! If you're really brave, enjoy this activity outside in the sun!

Oh, and remember, you are planting seeds. So, unless you want to be harvesting nine months from now, make sure you use some protection!

Working Overtime

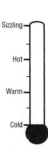

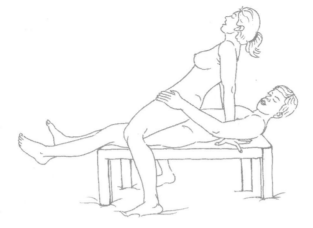

This position requires a piece of furniture, like a desk, where the woman's legs can hang over the sides. So clear off all those memos, legal pads, folders, and pencils. You have something much more interesting for her in-tray!

The man lies on his back with his legs spread open. Ladies, straddle your partner facing his feet. Lean backward resting your weight on your arms behind you. If your feet can touch the floor, use the leverage to help with the thrusting.

This position has a unique angle of penetration. As we have seen before, when the woman is leaning backward, the vagina expands to allow for deeper penetration. What makes this position unique is that the woman's legs are hanging over the edge of the furniture. The weight of her legs will pull down on her vaginal muscles. This changes the angle of penetration and also makes the vagina feel much tighter.

Working from home will take on a whole new meaning!

A Fresh Perspective

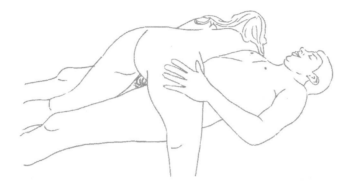

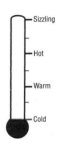

The woman on top in this position will definitely be seeing things from a different point of view! The new angle will feel a lot different too!

The man lies on his back with his legs out straight in front of him. The woman is lying on her tummy on top of her partner at a 45 degree angle to his head. Her legs are extended straight behind her and her arms should be flat on the bed in front of her.

The resulting angle of penetration is superb! It's different from the standard woman-on-top positions, but not exactly sideways penetration either. Very tight and very exhilarating!

Ladies, your pubic bone is resting on the man's hips. Each time you thrust your hips, make sure that your clitoris is stimulated. Gyrate your hips around looking for the spot that gives the best friction. Not only does this help you orgasm, it feels

great to your partner too!

Guys, knead your partner's buttocks with your hands. Push and pull the skin with your fingers and thumbs. Play a little drumbeat on it, slapping it gently. When you can feel her reaching her peak, push her hips down into yours to intensify her orgasm.

Both of you will be seeing and feeling things in a whole new way!

Blowing Your Top

Sizzling —

Hot —

Warm —

Cold —

Ladies, you do the blowing, but I don't think it's his top that will be exploding in this fellatio position.

Lie on your tummy with your head and shoulders at the edge of the bed. Have your partner stand next to the bed. Grab your partner around the legs and pull his hips to your face. Put just the head of his penis into your mouth and whip your tongue around the edges of it. Flatten your tongue and slide it all around the entire surface.

Open your mouth wide enough so that your partner can thrust his penis inside. Let him go as deep as you want, taking as much of his penis into your mouth as possible. Keep your lips sealed around the shaft of the penis while your partner thrusts his hips forward and backward. Flick your tongue around different areas on the shaft each time the penis is thrust forward. He'll love watching his penis glide in and out of your mouth!

Let your partner control the pace for this one. You'll see a volcanic eruption that rivals Mount Vesuvius!

Riding Shotgun

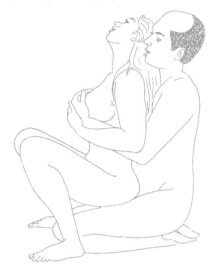

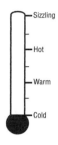

The woman is in the passenger's seat, but the man has got the shotgun!

Guys, kneel on the bed with your legs completely bent so that your bottom is resting on the backs of your calves, and your thighs are nice and flat. Lower your partner down into your lap, sliding your shotgun into her holster at the same time.

Ladies, sit on your partner's lap facing away from him. Bend your legs so that your feet are flat on the floor next to his knees. Your knees will be up by your chest. Spread your legs apart as wide as you can. This allows for the deepest penetration, but even more importantly, gives you lots of room to masturbate.

Guys, reach around to the front of your lover and take her breasts into your hands. Spread your fingers apart and use the whole hand to cover as much of the breast as possible. Massage them, pulling your fingers up from the base to the nipple. Tickle the palms of your hands with her taut nipples. Press your hands down, flattening her breasts, and rub them with your palms in a circular motion. Let your fingers explore, tickle, and massage the entire breast.

Get behind the wheel? No thanks. I prefer to ride shotgun!

Chip on Your Shoulder

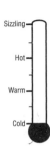

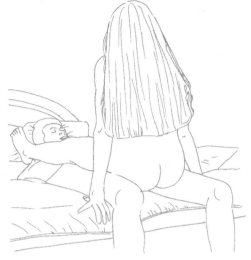

Lie on your back, guys, with your legs hanging over the edge of the bed. Push off the floor with your feet to get the best thrusting.

Gals, sit on top of your partner, but in front of his penis. Spread your legs open wide. While your partner is watching, slip your finger into your vagina. Pull it back out and rub it all around, lubricating the entire vaginal area. Guys find this incredibly erotic! Do it once or twice more and then close your legs.

When you're good and ready, lift yourself up and move backward so that you are positioned above the man's penis. Wrap your hand around the shaft and give it a few strokes while you guide the head to your vagina and allow penetration. Put your legs straight out in front of you so that they are resting on your partner's shoulders. Squeeze your feet together, locking his penis in a vaginal embrace and his head in a leg embrace. Feel his thrusts deep inside of you as he reaches his peak.

Burning the Midnight Oil

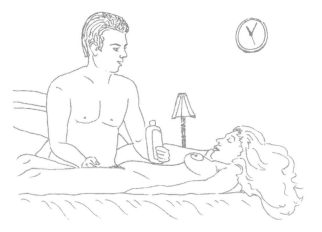

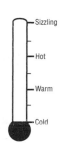

Guys, you'll need some oil or lotion for this activity. Be creative and try something new. Your choices are almost endless!

There are oils, lotions, and creams. You'll have to experiment with some of each to figure out what you like best. Some people think that oils are too sticky. Others find that lotions are not slippery enough. You'll only learn which you prefer by sampling a variety of them.

Lotions, oils, and creams also come in a wide variety of scents and colors. The edible oils are even flavored. Pick a scent you think your partner will like. Some women like fruity sweet scents. Others prefer a soapy or flowery scent. One scent might be relaxing; another scent will be stimulating. Again, only by experimenting will you figure out which products work best for each mood and scenario.

So, you've picked out a lotion, oil, or cream. Pour some into your hands and rub it into your partner's skin. Massage her breasts and nipples with it. Pour some down her tummy and rub it into her skin with your hands. Rub it all over her legs. Using your slippery fingers, manually stimulate her clitoris. Some of the oils will increase the clitoral sensations. Bring your partner to a full and deep orgasm.

Here's a little extra suggestion. Now is a great time to engage in intercourse. Her skin is slick and smooth. Choose a position with lots of skin-to-skin contact and slide around together!

Old Friend

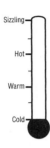

Sizzling

Hot

Warm

Cold

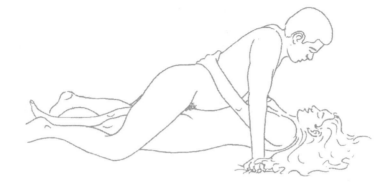

Tonight's position is one that virtually everyone has used at least once, and most people have probably used frequently. Tonight's position is the standard man-on-top missionary position. After all the variety of the last few months, this position is like returning to an old friend. It's comfortable and familiar. And while it might not be the most exciting position in the book, a sex book really is not complete without it.

Pay extra attention tonight to the small, warm, loving details of intercourse. Remind your partner about the things you love the most about them. Tell them how much you appreciate all the great things they do. Let them know that your life is better because they are part of it. And afterward, thank them for being a wonderful person and, of course, a willing sex partner!

The Organ Grinder

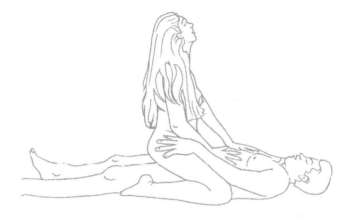

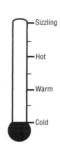

Sizzling

Hot

Warm

Cold

Crank the shaft and this organ will produce some beautiful music!

The man lies on his back with his legs out straight in front of him. The shaft of his organ should be in an upright position for cranking.

Ladies, sit on top of your partner with your legs bent so that your feet are behind you. Spread your legs apart as far as possible so that you can rub your pubic bone up against your partner's pelvis.

You get to be the organ grinder! Gyrate your hips and grind them down, rubbing your clitoris against your partner. Move from side to side, forward and backward, and around in a circle. Let your partner do the thrusting while you play your own song on the organ. Let the interlude build to a resounding duet crescendo!

Heads or Tails?

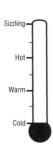

Sizzling

Hot

Warm

Cold

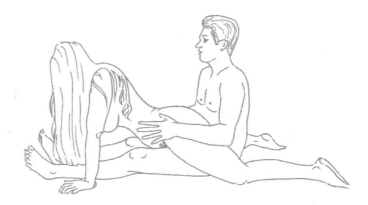

Looks like tails to me!

The man sits on the bed with his legs straight in front of him. Ladies, facing his feet, straddle your partner with your legs by his hips and your hands by his feet. Let your partner guide your hips to the tip of his penis, then lower yourself down the shaft. His head should be so deep that your tail is pushing into his stomach!

Guys, grab your partner's hips and slide them up and down the shaft of your penis. Use your hands to massage her buttocks and thighs. Tell your partner she's been naughty and gently spank her bottom. Separate her cheeks and use your finger to stimulate the sensitive areas around her rectum. Many women find this powerfully arousing!

Heads or tails? His head and her tail. It's a winning coin toss every time.

All-You-Can-Eat Special

Month 4
Day 16

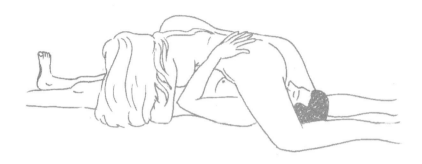

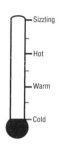

And, tonight it's two for the price of one!

Start the night out with a shower together. Many people find oral sex much more attractive and fun when their partner is extra clean.

Ladies, straddle your partner so that your hips are over his face and your face is over his hips.

Now both of you can dig into your meal!

Guys, pull your partner's hips down to your face. Latch your mouth around her entire clitoral area,

surrounding it with a warm, wet, and wonderful sensation! Rub your tongue around on her clitoris. Use a variety of techniques to keep things unpredictable. Sometimes have the tongue pointed; at other times have it flat. Sometimes rub the tongue in circles; at other times rub it back and forth. When she clenches your face with her thighs, you'll know she's nearly to the point of orgasm!

Ladies, lower your mouth onto your partner's penis,

letting it go as deep as possible. Lift and lower your head, allowing his penis to slide in and out of your mouth without losing penetration. Flick your tongue around the head of the penis, particularly along the slit in the back. You're stimulating a very sensitive area that will keep him wanting more! Increase the pace until he orgasms.

The all-you-can-eat special is good for the whole night. Keep satisfying your hunger again and again!

Golfer's Delight

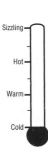

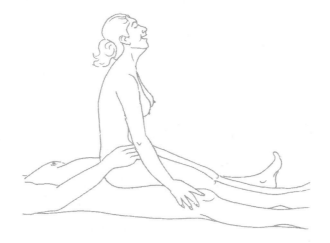

This golf course will satisfy golfers of all abilities. But first, you need the right equipment. This hole requires a long club with a strong shaft. A woody tends to work better than an iron. And, always play with two balls.

Guys, lie down on your back with your legs spread out wide in front you. Your partner will be sitting on your lap, facing your feet. Line up the hole with the club and hit your drive long and straight. You'll notice that the course feels a little wet. Don't worry! This will actually improve your game!

Ladies, you will be sitting on your partner's lap facing his feet. Your legs should be straight in front of you. The fairway on this hole is very narrow. It doesn't have a lot of trees, but it's got a great bush! Use your hand to take care of your partner's balls. Rolling them around in your hand and playing with them will improve his score. Bouncing them on the cart path, however, is not recommended!

Play as slow or as fast as you want, and use as many strokes as you need to finish the hole.

Who needs a hole-in-one when you can have one in the hole?

Bake at 350 Degrees

Month 4
Day 18

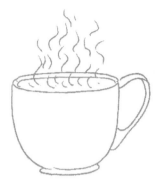

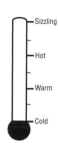

This is a cunnilingus activity that is sure to get her oven hot!

Guys, get a coffee cup full of steaming hot water or coffee. Have your partner lie down on the bed with her legs spread wide open. Being careful not to burn your tongue, either hold your tongue against the warm cup or hold some of the hot coffee on your tongue for a few seconds. Then, immediately (well, after setting the cup back down) lower your tongue onto your lover's clitoris. The extra warmth greatly intensifies the sensations! For some women, this single movement will be enough to induce a small orgasm!

Warm your tongue again and lick around the vagina. Again, the heat will drive her wild! Apply your warmed tongue to her labia, closing the lips to seal in the heat. Finally, use your tongue to rub back and forth on her clitoris to bring her to a full orgasm.

Baking times vary depending on the oven. Do not overbake!

Easy Come, Easy Go!

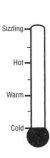

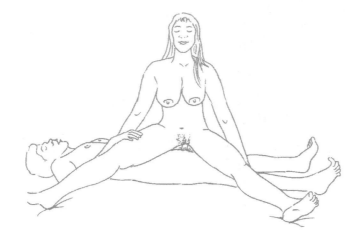

This is a very easy position to master!

Ladies, have your partner lie on his back with his legs out straight. Sit on top of your partner facing sideways. Spread your legs wide open in front of you.

After penetration, thrust your hips forward and backward. Remember that since you're sitting sideways, this will feel like side-to-side thrusting to your partner. It's very tight and very pleasant. Circle your hips around a bit as you grind into his hips. Keep things interesting. Move forward and backward, side to side, and around in a circle. He'll think it all feels great!

And, ladies, don't leave yourself out of this one. With your legs spread wide open, this position is a masturbator's dream! Use your fingers or a vibrator!

Come one, come all for this position!

Blind Date

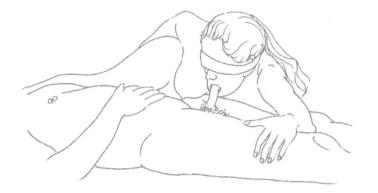

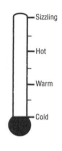

This is a blindfolded fellatio activity with a little twist. It's not the guy that gets blindfolded; it's the woman! So, ladies, tie a scarf over your eyes. And no peeking!

Put your hands behind your back, gals. Even blindfolded, this activity is much too easy if you can use your hands! Lean over and find your partner with your face and head. Rub up against him to figure out which body part you're touching and which direction you need to be moving. Work your way to his groin and stroke his penis against your face.

Without using your hand to hold it still, lower your mouth over the head of your partner's penis. Don't be surprised if you miss the first time. Or maybe even the second time. Use your tongue, mouth, and fellatio skills to stimulate your partner to orgasm.

You might feel a bit clumsy and awkward without your hands or eyes, but have fun! Fellatio is an old activity. Doing it blindfolded and without hands makes it feel new and interesting again. So, ladies, have a good laugh. And remember, your partner will be blindfolded for a cunnilingus activity later this year!

Geometry Lesson

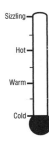

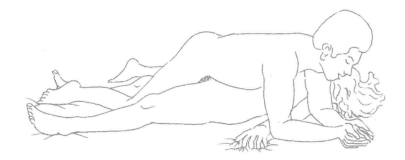

Get out your protractor because we've got some angles to measure!

Guys, have your partner lie flat on her back. Lie down on top of her so that your body is at a 45 degree angle to her body. To help spread her legs apart, have one of her legs entwined between your legs. Bend your arms in front of you so that you can rest your weight on your elbows.

Penetration can be a little tricky with this position. If you try to rush it, your penis will be poking up against your partner's pelvis bone. It's not very deep and it doesn't feel very pleasant for either of you! So go slowly. Turn your hips so your penis is pointing in the direction of the woman's vagina. After carefully sliding your penis inside, turn your hips back so that

they are at a 45 degree angle again. Now when you thrust, it will feel wonderfully tight as you push your penis head into the side of her vagina.

An angle is the space between two lines that diverge from a single point. Funny, we never studied lines as interesting as these or single points that were this hot when I was in geometry class!

Full Moon Rising

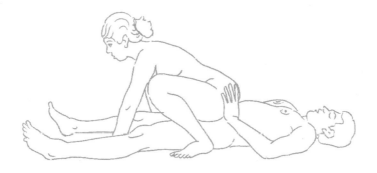

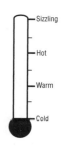

Sizzling

Hot

Warm

Cold

You don't need to do this one at night to see the full moon. The moon can be seen even in the middle of the day!

The man lies on his back with his legs straight in front of him. Ladies, sit on top of your partner facing his feet. Your legs should be bent and your feet should be flat on the floor next to the man's hips. This feels a lot like squatting.

After penetration, lean forward, putting your weight on your arms in front of you. Remember to lean slowly because you'll be bending your partner's penis to an angle that is contrary to how it usually hangs. By leaning, you significantly tighten the penetration.

Guys, as your partner leans forward, watch her full moon rise. You get a great view of her entire back end! Firmly massage her buttocks with your hands. If you're feeling a little playful or naughty, spank her bottom.

Have your partner sit up and lean forward again. Who says a full moon can only occur once every thirty days?

Knee Pads Optional

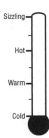

Sizzling

Hot

Warm

Cold

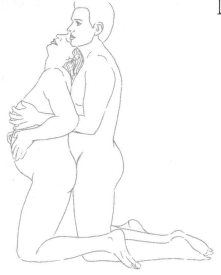

This is a rear-entry position with both of you on your knees. So if you have rough carpeting or a hardwood floor, you might want to consider some protective knee pads!

Ladies, kneel on the floor. This position is much easier if you have something like the bed or the wall to lean against. Have your partner kneel behind you with his legs between your legs.

Guys, the best way to get penetration is to lower your hips down far enough to guide the tip of your penis to the entrance of her vagina. Raise your hips, thrusting your penis inside at the same time. It's a tight fit, so be sure your partner is nice and wet before you penetrate.

Use one hand to reach around and manually stimulate your lover. Wrap your other hand around the base of your penis. Feel your penis slide in and out of your hand and her vagina as you thrust your hips back and forth. When you feel your partner reaching her climax, tighten the grip on your penis so that you can reach your peak at the same time.

Finger Painting

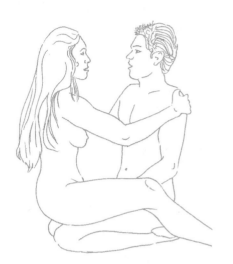

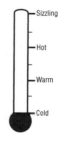

Sizzling

Hot

Warm

Cold

Guys, this is a position where you get to manually stimulate your partner. Kneel down on the bed. Have your partner sit down on your lap making sure that she's not too close. You need to leave enough room for your hand.

Use the finger painting techniques you learned in elementary school to stimulate your partner. Use the side of your hand to paint long strokes up and down her labia. With several fingers, paint large circles around the clitoral area from the top of one thigh to the other. Use your fingertips to very lightly brush from side to side. Circle your fingers around the clitoris. Finish your painting by firmly rubbing your fingers back and forth over her clitoris.

Your partner will think you've created a masterpiece.

Naughty Is Sooooo Nice!

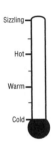

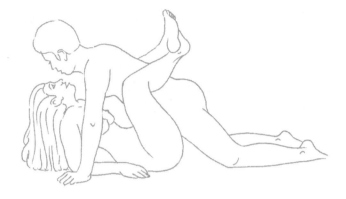

Lie on your back, ladies, with your arms bent and your weight resting on your elbows. After your partner has penetrated, wrap your legs tightly around his waist.

Guys, kneel down between your partner's legs. Lean forward with your weight on your arms. Lower your lips to your partner's ear and tell her all the naughty things you plan to do. But remember, talking dirty is not the same as being vulgar! Most women are not interested in being called derogatory names or hearing excessively crude sexual descriptions. Women like it when their men are sensual and sexy.

Insert your finger into her vagina and tell her how warm and moist she is. Tell her you can't wait to be deep inside of her. Lower your hips, sliding your penis into her vagina. Let her know how tight she is and how great it feels to be stroking in and out. Tell her that you want to make her come.

You get the idea. Talk dirty, but be creative and sensual. Tell her explicit details, but avoid hard-core locker room talk. Emphasize the positives about your partner, the sex, and the orgasm.

Pleasant Dreams

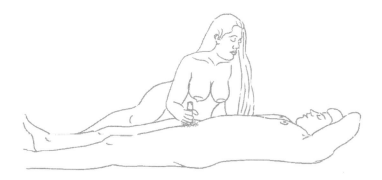

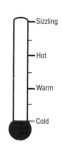

Sizzling

Hot

Warm

Cold

Okay, ladies, time to give your partner some very pleasant dreams!

This activity will be done after your partner is sound asleep. Women whose lovers fall asleep quickly and easily can do this within a few minutes after going to bed. Other women may have to save this activity and use it when they wake up during the middle of the night.

If your partner is lying on his stomach, pull the covers or jostle him a bit to get him to roll over onto his back or side. Reach down and wrap your hand around his penis. Some of you will be surprised to find that he's already erect! Rub your hand up and down the shaft. He'll respond, even in his sleep! Lengthen the stroke to include both the shaft and the head of the penis. At some point, the sensations become too strong for him to sleep through. He'll wake up to a few seconds of confusion followed by an overwhelming sensation of warmth, arousal, and stimulation. Men find it incredibly erotic to wake up to their partner masturbating them! Continue stroking your partner until he orgasms.

This activity will remind him that dreams really can come true!

Take a Bow

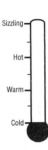

Sizzling

Hot

Warm

Cold

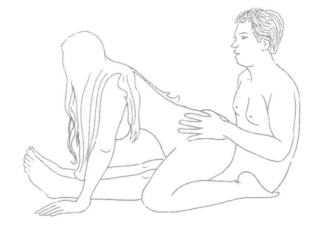

Ladies, have your partner sit on the bed with his legs straight in front of him. Sit on your partner's lap facing his feet. Your legs should be bent so that your feet are behind you.

Once penetration has occurred, lean your upper body forward. This will elevate your hips and give you a great opportunity to rub your bottom into your partner's torso. Bow forward as far as you can. According to ancient custom, the lower the bow, the more respect that is being shown. In this case, the lower the bow, the tighter the penetration will be.

This position is great for stimulating the front vaginal wall, home of the elusive G-spot. As you thrust your hips up and down your lover's shaft, move your hips around until you find a sensitive spot that gets stimulated by the head of his penis. Increase the pace of your thrusts until both of you have climaxed.

Then, stand up, take a bow, and enjoy your partner's applause!

Diddly Squat

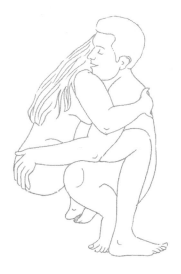

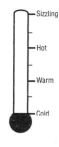

Hope you've been doing your deep knee bends because this position requires a little leg strength!

For this position, both of you will be squatting. Guys, you should squat first. Your legs can be spread apart or kept together depending on what feels comfortable. Get your feet comfortable and your weight distributed evenly. If you're unbalanced, you'll fall over when your partner gets on top!

Ladies, face your partner and squat over his legs. Use your hands to insert his penis as you lower yourself down to his thighs. Try to keep most of your weight on your feet rather than resting it on your partner's lap. He'll be grateful for this!

This position is perfect for holding each other tight. Maximize the amount of skin-to-skin contact. Take turns using your strong leg muscles to thrust by lifting and lowering yourself.

Skip your workout at the gym. This is a much more rewarding exercise!

Tongue-tied

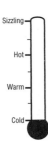

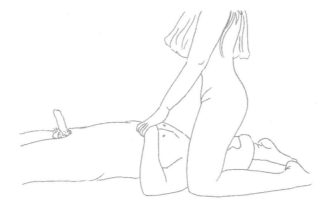

Your tongue will be too busy during this cunnilingus position to do much talking!

Ladies, kneel down on the bed straddling your partner's face. You should be facing your partner's feet. Spread your legs apart wide so that your pelvis is low enough for your partner to reach with his mouth. If it feels comfortable, lean forward and rub your breasts against your partner's torso. It's very stimulating for him, and feels good for you too!

Guys, lie on your back with a few pillows under your head. Grasp your partner's hips and lower her to your face. Point your tongue and firmly run it up and down her labia all the way from her clitoris to her vagina and back. Lick the skin between the vagina and her anus. This is an extremely sensitive area that is often ignored. Work your way back up to her clitoris. Roll your tongue around the entire clitoral area. Position your mouth around the clitoris and rub your tongue back and forth. Enjoy the sensation of her hips grinding into your face as you bring her to orgasm.

Split Personality

Month 4
Day 30

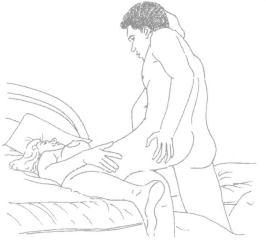

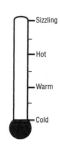

Sizzling

Hot

Warm

Cold

Lie on your back, ladies, with your legs hanging over the edge of the bed. Make sure your hips are all the way to the edge of the bed so that the man can easily penetrate. Start by having both feet on the floor. Once your partner has penetrated, split your legs by lifting one up and moving it to his shoulder.

Guys, your legs are also split. One knee is resting on the bed holding most of your weight. The other leg is bent with the knee on the floor. Because of the leg on the bed, you can get very deep penetration.

Encourage your partner to masturbate. You'll feel her hand bumping against your pelvic bone each time you thrust. You'll find it very pleasant!

All personalities will love this position!

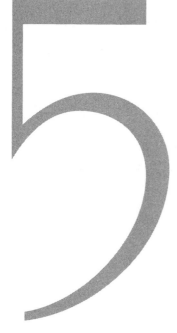

MONTH 5

Day 1. Flashback

Day 2. Smoking Gun

Day 3. Is It Hot or Is It Just Me?

Day 4. The Midas Touch

Day 5. Hold It Right There!

Day 6. Laying Down the Law

Day 7. The Catbird Seat

Day 8. Blowing Your Load

Day 9. Speaking in Tongues

Day 10. Laid to Rest

Day 11. Bending Over Backward

Day 12. Space Mission

Day 13. Is That My Pager?

Day 14. Nuts and Bolts

Day 15. Blow Your Own Horn

Day 16. Sit Tight

Day 17. Raise the Flag

Day 18. Totally Titillating

Day 19. Taking Care of Business

Day 20. In the Doghouse

Day 21. Get a Grip

Day 22. Knock Her Socks Off

Day 23. Skin and Boners

Day 24. Standing Room Only

Day 25. Reflections

Day 26. Choosing Sides

Day 27. Whipped Cream and Nuts

Day 28. Back in the Saddle Again

Day 29. Neck and Neck

Day 30. Bottom Feeder

Flashback

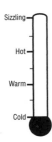

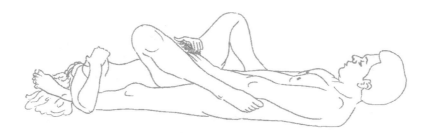

Get ready to go to the moon and back! This position has both of you on your backs. So put on a little background music and get back to basics.

Ladies, have your partner lie flat on his back. You will start by sitting on your partner facing him. Your legs should be completely bent so that your feet are by your partner's hips. Once your partner is deep inside of you, reach your hand behind you and give his testicles a little backspin. Then, slowly lean backward until your back is against his legs.

Guys, you are back in control for this one. Use your backhand to do a little backstroke on your lover's clitoris. Rub it back and forth. Tease her a bit. Arouse her, then back off, then arouse her again. Once her hips start thrusting, there's no looking back. Take this one to a climactic finish.

Don't put this position on the back burner. Mark the page so you can keep coming back.

Smoking Gun

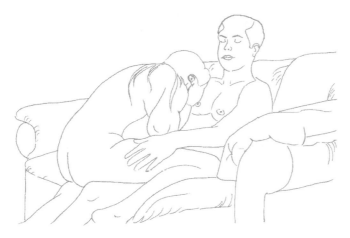

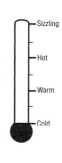

Sign up for the firearms training class, ladies. This is a position where you will be manually stimulating your partner.

Have the Top Gun sit comfortably in a chair. You will be sitting in his lap facing him. Get your partner in your sights and put your fingers on his trigger. Use your hand to stroke up and down the shaft of his penis. Start nice and slow. Save the rapid-fire speed for when he's closer to orgasm.

Lean forward to lick and suck on your partner's nipples. Men find this very stimulating! Sit close enough to your partner that you can rub his penis around on your clitoris. Let him feel the heat, but don't let him in the bullet hole. Rub your hand up and down the shaft, steadily increasing the pace, until all of his ammunition has been fired.

Is It Hot or Is It Just Me?

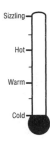

Sizzling

Hot

Warm

Cold

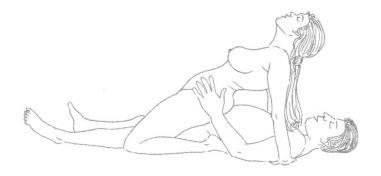

It's hot! Very hot!

For this position, the man lies on his back with his legs straight out in front of him. The woman sits on top facing the man's feet. Her legs should be bent so that her feet are behind her.

Ladies, after penetration, put your arms behind you and lean back. Feel how much deeper he can thrust now. If your hair is long enough, lean your head back and let your hair drape across his chest. Swish it slowly from side to side across his nipples. The hair is so light. It produces a wonderful tickling feeling that can't be duplicated with fingers.

Shift your weight so you are leaning on just one arm. Use your other hand to masturbate. Let your partner know how great it feels when he's thrusting deep inside of you. Raise and lower your hips to make his thrusts even more powerful. Push your hips down into his pelvis as both of you orgasm.

Is it hot in here or is it just me?

The Midas Touch

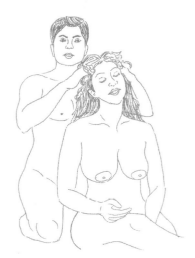

Sizzling

Hot

Warm

Cold

Guys: Tonight you are the king with the golden touch. And you'll be doing lots of touching! This is a massage activity that culminates with manual stimulation to your lover's clitoris.

Let's start at the top. Begin by scratching your partner's scalp with your fingernails. Women love this! It feels particularly good down by the neckline. Massage your way from her neck down to her pubic hair. Be sure to include her arms, shoulders, breasts, and stomach.

A good massage will use a variety of techniques. Sometimes your hands should be completely flat. This is great for large areas like the chest or stomach. Keep all the fingers spread apart and push your hands forward in long, gentle strokes. Pull up a fold of skin and knead it between your fingers and thumbs. In some areas, like arms, shoulders, and breasts, use your full hand in a kneading motion, working the skin with the heel of your hand.

Alter the pressure as you move your hands. Kneading uses a firm grasp on the skin. Follow this up by delicately brushing over the skin with your fingertips. Tickle the skin with your fingernails in places like the inside of her arms. Try not to be predictable. Randomly change whether you are using hard pressure, soft pressure, or something in between.

After your partner is tingling all over from the wonderful massage, work your way to her pubic hair. Rub your hand through her pubic hair and gently pull it. Keep your hand in her pubic hair while your fingertips start rubbing back and forth on her clitoris. Use your other hand to stimulate her vagina. Insert a finger, or two, and mimic the feeling of penetration. A good orgasm is worth its weight in gold!

Hold It Right There!

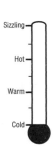

Sizzling
Hot
Warm
Cold

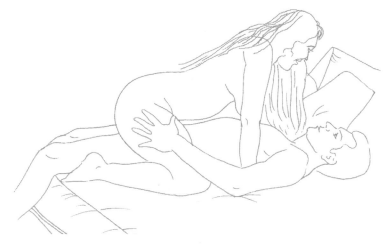

This position is so great for holding your partner! I'm sure they'll let you know exactly where they want to be held!

Ladies, have your partner lie on his back with his legs hanging over the edge of the bed. You'll be on top for this position, so straddle your lover facing him. Bend your legs with your feet behind you. Start with your legs bent just enough so that your hips can hover over the head of his penis. Lower your hips enough so that just the tip of the penis is inserted. Then completely bend your knees and slide smoothly down the shaft.

Lean all the way forward toward your lover. Hold his face in your hands and kiss his eyes, nose, cheeks, and lips. Whisper nice things about him in his ears.

Guys, put your arms around your lover and hold her very tight. Feel her breasts being pushed into your chest. Stroke your hands up and down her lower back. Use your legs to thrust nice and deep. Hold her right there as you reach your peak.

Laying Down the Law

Month 5
Day 6

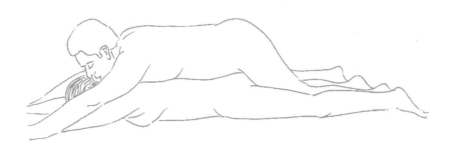

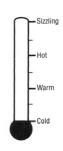

Sizzling
Hot
Warm
Cold

A fugitive from your love is on the loose and needs to be apprehended. Use caution! She has arms and is seductively dangerous! When you spot her, point your loaded gun at her and instruct her to lie down on her stomach with her hands over her head.

Kneel down between your partner's legs. Pat her down from head to toe searching for weapons. Do a background check. Massage her buttocks with your hands. Spread her cheeks apart and rub your fingers between them. Gently tickle the area around her rectum. Don't worry about leaving fingerprints.

Bend down even further to insert the tip of your penis into your lover's vagina. Slide your penis all the way in as you lower yourself on top of her. This is a repeat offender. Definitely hold her without bail. Thrust your hips forward and backward until both of you are seeing flashing lights and wailing like sirens!

After she's served her time, let her go free!

The Catbird Seat

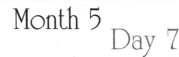

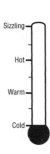

Sizzling

Hot

Warm

Cold

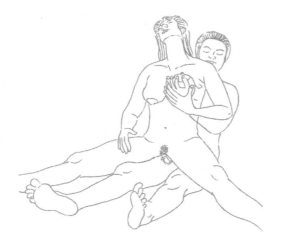

Exactly who has the catbird seat for this position? Is it the woman because she's got the higher, more dominant perch? Or is it the man, who has a warm fuzzy cat sitting on his nest? Try it out and decide for yourself!

The man sits with his legs straight out in front of him. The woman sits on the man's lap facing outward toward the man's feet. Her legs should be spread open wide.

Guys, you've got two free hands and your lover sitting in your lap in front of you.

No need to kill many brain cells trying to figure out what to do! Reach around and put your hands squarely on her breasts. Spread your fingers and massage as much of her breast as you can hold. Lift your hand and drag your fingers to her nipple. Gently squeeze her nipple between your thumb and finger. It produces a very sharp and arousing sensation!

Ladies, use one hand to masturbate while you thrust and grind your hips.

Use your other hand to fondle your partner's testicles. As you approach orgasm, move your hand from his testicles to the base of his penis and grasp it tightly. This extra surge of stimulation will help him reach his peak simultaneously with you.

So, who was in the catbird seat? If you can't come to an agreement, and you probably won't, try the position again for a second opinion!

Blowing Your Load

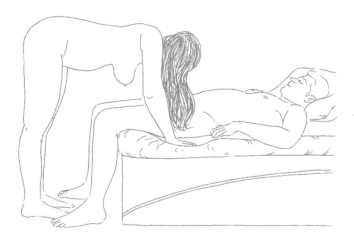

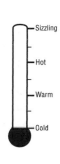

Sizzling

Hot

Warm

Cold

A fellatio position where she blows him and he blows his load!

Ladies, have your partner lie on the bed with his legs hanging over the edge. You will be standing next to the bed between his legs.

Start by bending over and dragging your hair across his stomach, penis, and thighs. It creates a very light, silky, delicate feeling that pleasantly tickles and sets the nerves on edge.

Kiss the very tip of your partner's penis. Flatten your tongue and lick all over the head. Run your tongue around the head where it meets the penis shaft. Enclose the entire head of the penis in your red-hot mouth.

Bend over further to lower your mouth around your lover's entire penis. Firmly seal your lips around the shaft. Rhythmically move your head up and down, letting the shaft of the penis slide in and out of your mouth. Keep the tongue moving around as much as possible. Feeling their lover's tongue rubbing up, down, and around on their penis is the favorite part of fellatio for many men.

Increase the heat and the intensity until your partner has blown his load!

Speaking in Tongues

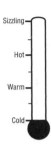

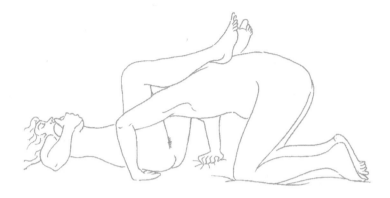

And, guys, your tongue has a lot to say! Of course, it won't be using many words during this cunnilingus position.

Ladies, lie on your back with your legs spread open. After your partner has knelt down between your legs, put your legs around his shoulders or neck and give him a tight leg embrace. His face will be locked between your legs. You just can't ask

for much more!

Guys, get your tongue ready to do some talking. Start by kissing and stroking her inner thigh. Your lips and fingers should barely touch her skin. It's a tease, and it works!

Using your fingers to spread apart her labia, point your tongue and lick the skin around the clitoris. Use a short, probing stroke that applies pressure to a very

small area with each lick. Steadily lengthen the stroke and increase the amount of tongue that touches your partner's skin. Eventually, flatten the tongue and press it up against her clitoris. Speak the language of orgasm by firmly licking back and forth across her clitoris.

Your partner might be speaking in tongues too. Some feelings are just too good for words!

Laid to Rest

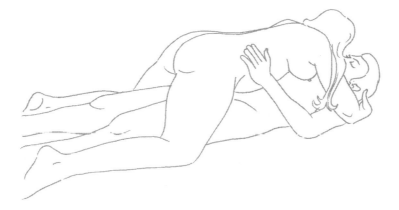

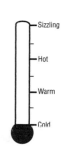

Sizzling

Hot

Warm

Cold

The French phrase for orgasm is *le petit mort*, which means "the little death." Thankfully, for most of us, even the best sex isn't enough to send us to the big bedroom in the sky.

For this position, the man lies on his back with his legs out straight. The woman lies on top of the man facing him. Her legs should be spread open behind her.

This is a very loving and intimate position. Guys, put your arms around your lover and hold her close as she moves up and down. Whisper quietly to each other. Nibble on your partner's ears and neck. Passionately kiss each other. Enjoy the skin-on-skin contact. Feel the heat being generated by your partner as their arousal climaxes with an orgasm.

Your loving partner. Great sex. Maybe you did die and go to heaven!

Bending Over Backward

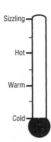

Sizzling

Hot

Warm

Cold

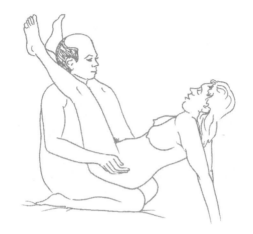

Trying to find that elusive G-spot? This position may be the answer!

The man kneels on the bed with his legs completely bent. Ladies, using one hand to guide your partner's penis to your vagina, sit down on your partner's lap with your feet down on the bed. Put your arms behind you and lean backward.

Finally, lift your legs up onto your partner's shoulders.

As your partner thrusts, the head of his penis will be bumping up against the front wall of your vagina, where the G-spot lies waiting to be discovered. With the weight of your upper body resting on your arms, move your hips up and down the shaft of your partner's penis. Experiment with deep and shallow penetration, until you find a depth that is particularly stimulating. Have your partner use his hand to manually stimulate your clitoris at the same time. Experience an orgasm that takes your breath away!

Space Mission

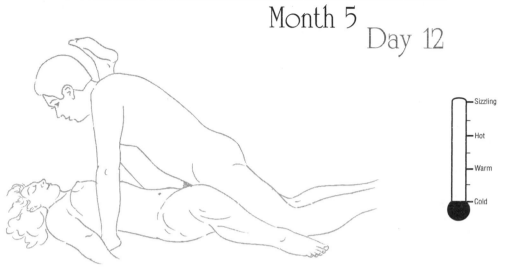

Sizzling

Hot

Warm

Cold

Get ready to blast off into outer space. Good astronomers will be seeing lots of stars!

This is a variation of the standard missionary position. The woman is on her back, but her legs are not straight out in front of her. One leg is bent so that her foot is up by her bottom. The other leg is up on her partner's shoulder.

Guys, this position is very deep! Start your space exploration by inserting your telescope into her black hole. Feel the heat of her sun as you explore your lover's universe. Look down and enjoy the terrific view of two beautiful planets. Make eye contact with your partner. Let her know that she is the center of your galaxy.

Probe your telescope deeper and deeper until both of you experience an astronomical explosion of shooting stars!

Is That My Pager?

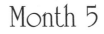

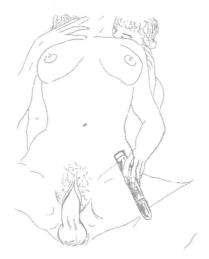

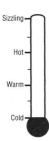

Sizzling
Hot
Warm
Cold

You'll feel a vibration, but it definitely is not your pager!

Ladies, this is an activity where you use the vibrator to stimulate your partner during intercourse. Pick a position where you have access to the man's testicles. A position where you sit on top of your partner facing his feet works great for this. If you need help finding a position for this activity, try one of those suggested below.

After penetration, start up the vibrator. Using the vibrator greatly magnifies the intensity of the stimulation. So don't move to his genitals until you're ready for him to climax. Rub it along his thighs from his knee to the very top of the inner thigh. Use the vibrator on his chest and arms if you can reach them. Eventually, hold the vibrator up against his testicles. This is an incredibly powerful sensation! If you can, put the vibrator up against the base of his penis. Let it touch his penis as he thrusts in and out of you. Enjoy feeling him thrust deep inside of you as he reaches an explosive peak.

Set his pager to vibrate. Each time it goes off, he'll be thinking of you and some very erotic memories!

Suggested Positions: Month 2/Day 3 — Great Balls of Fire; Month 5/Day 14 — Nuts and Bolts; Month 6/Day 5 — Flagpole Sitting; Month 7/Day 16 — Looking Forward to This; Month 11/Day 4 — Follow the Bouncing Ball.

Nuts and Bolts

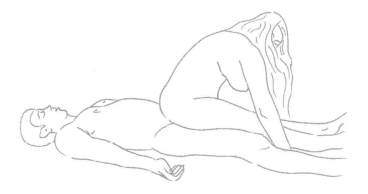

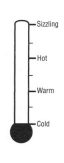

You'll go nuts over this position!

Ladies, have your partner lie on his back with his legs spread apart. Be sure that his nuts are accessible and his bolt is upright. Use your mouth to get your partner's penis wet and lubricated. Sit down on top of your partner facing his feet, and put your legs straight in front of you. This results in a very tight and snug penetration.

Lean all the way forward and simultaneously reach down between your partner's legs and wrap your hand around his nuts. Squeeze them. Massage them. Gently tug on them. Roll them around between your fingers. Do whatever comes to mind to make them feel great! Every move you make on the nuts will have a direct effect on the bolt! Lift and lower your hips as your partner thrusts. As your partner approaches his peak, squeeze your vaginal muscles firmly together to intensify the pleasure of his orgasm.

Blow Your Own Horn

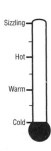

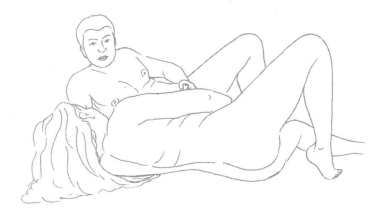

This is a do-it-yourself dual masturbation position. Unlike some animals, humans are not able to literally blow their own horns. So, use your hand instead!

Watching your partner masturbate can be both stimulating and educational. Sometimes, we learn little tricks about what our partner likes by watching how they stimulate themselves.

Lie next to each other on the bed, facing each other. Each of you should use one hand to masturbate. Put the other hand on your partner's hand as they masturbate. This gives you each one hand on the bottom that you control and one hand on the top that your partner controls.

Explore each other's bodies by moving around the hand that you control. Show your partner where and how you like to be touched. Keep your partner's hand with you as you manually stimulate your own genitals. Take turns masturbating. When it's your partner's turn, let your fingers get a lesson on how to please. When it's your turn, show your partner your favorite technique to bring you to orgasm.

Not ready for the music to end? Now that each of you has taught your partner your favorite song, let your partner play it for you!

Sit Tight

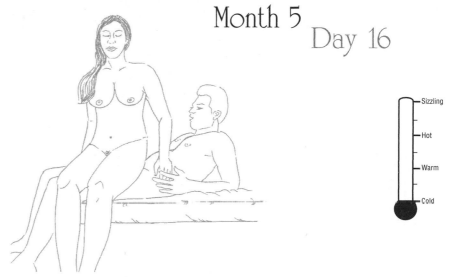

Sizzling

Hot

Warm

Cold

And, it's very tight!

Guys, lie on your back with your legs hanging over the edge of the bed. Bend your arms behind you and rest your weight on your elbows. This elevates your head and shoulders, and gives you a much better view!

Ladies, you'll be sitting on your partner's lap facing away from him. To make

penetration easier, spread your legs apart. Have your partner hold his penis steady while you line up your hips and lower yourself down his shaft.

Make the penetration as tight as you can. Move your legs so that both of them are on the same side of your partner's legs. Sideways penetration is always tight! Push your legs together as

close as possible. This compresses the vagina. Contract and tighten your vaginal muscles. This causes a very noticeable difference in making the vagina feel smaller. Your partner will feel the difference immediately as you move up and down his penis.

Your partner wants to do this one again? Tell him to sit tight!

Raise the Flag

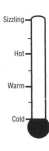

Sizzling —

Hot —

Warm —

Cold —

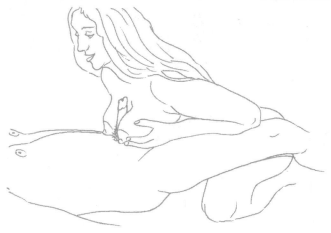

Ladies: This is a manual stimulation activity that is going to require some planning and premeditation because it starts while the penis is still limp. If your partner has an overactive libido, this activity might be impossible!

Men love how it feels to get hard in their lover's hand. It's a rush that can't be compared to any other aspect of sexual pleasure. So, wrap your hand around your partner's penis while it's soft, and very lightly start to stroke it. Unless he's comatose (and maybe even then), he'll start responding immediately! Take it slow. The buildup for this activity is as important as the peak.

Although this activity can also be done while the man sits in a chair or is standing, I recommend that you have your partner lie down on his back. Then, kneel down between his legs, lean over, and rub his penis between your breasts. Push your breasts together, leaving just enough room for your partner's penis to slide back and forth. Put a little oil or lotion on your breasts to make them extra slippery! Manually bring your partner to orgasm using either your hands or your breasts.

Be patriotic. Raise the flag and fly it often!

Totally Titillating

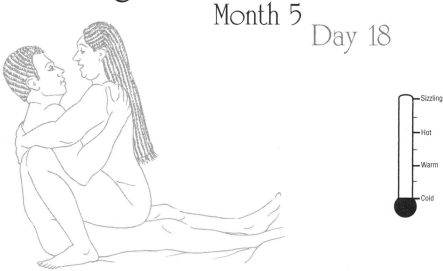

Sizzling

Hot

Warm

Cold

Did you ever notice that just saying the word titillate makes you feel a little tingly? Well, this titillating position will make you feel very tingly!

Guys, sit on the bed with your legs out straight in front of you. Have your partner sit on your lap facing you. Her legs should be bent so that her feet are next to

your hips. After penetration, titillate her. Place your hands on her breasts. With your palms over the nipples, use your fingers to massage and knead the sides. Push her breasts together and nuzzle your face into the cleavage. Rub the nipple back and forth between your thumb and finger. Gently pull it and squeeze it.

When you start reaching your peak, put your arms tightly around your partner and pull her to you. Rub her breasts into your chest as you orgasm.

Make a point to use the word titillate at least once in conversation tomorrow. If nothing else, it will remind you of what you had today!

Taking Care of Business

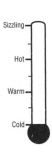

Sizzling

Hot

Warm

Cold

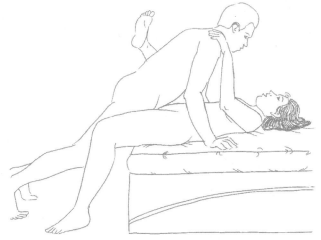

This is a business transaction that will be very profitable for both of you!

Ladies, lie down on your back with your legs hanging over the edge of the bed. Once your partner has penetrated, wrap one of your legs around his waist.

Guys, spread your lover's legs open and stand between them. Grasp your penis in your hand and lower your hips so that your penis can reach her vulva. Insert just the penis head into her vagina, getting it nice and wet. Use the head of your penis to spread the wetness to her labia. Dip back into the vagina again, and then rub around the clitoral area. Continue this until her entire vulva is wet and slippery.

Finally, insert the full length of your penis into your lover's vagina. Feel the moist heat that surrounds it, and the pleasant sensation of your lover's leg wrapped around your waist. After all that stimulation, this shop won't be open for business very long!

In the Doghouse

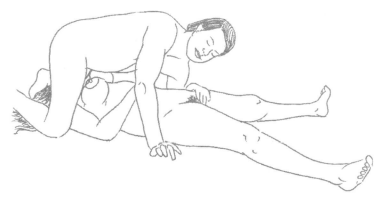

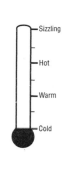

Sizzling

Hot

Warm

Cold

If you're in the doghouse, this position will get you out. If not, use this as a "Get Out of the Doghouse Free" card! You never know when you'll need it.

Ladies, lie on your back with your legs spread apart. Guys, facing her feet, get on your hands and knees and straddle your partner. Your hands should be by her hips. Your knees should be by her shoulders.

Balance your weight on one arm and use the other hand to manually stimulate your partner. If you normally stimulate your partner while kneeling between her legs, this position will give you a completely different angle. Rub the heel of your hand against her clitoris as you insert your finger into her vagina. Move your hand around in a circular motion. As you feel her clitoris swell beneath your hand, switch to a back-and-forth motion. Feel her vaginal muscles tighten around your finger as she climaxes.

Ladies, enjoy the view as your lover is straddled over you. Massage his buttocks. Stroke and tickle his anus. If you're a true dog lover, you'll throw him a bone. Grasp his penis and masturbate him after he has finished pleasing you. Or roll over and have intercourse. Use a doggy-style position, of course!

Get a Grip

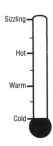

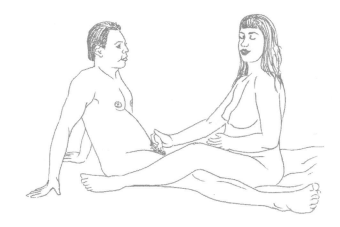

And, ladies, when it comes to manually stimulating your partner, you have a choice of which type of grip you want to get!

Have your partner sit on the bed with his legs spread wide open. Sit on his thighs with your legs around by his hips. Sit close, but leave enough space so that your hands can move about freely.

Tonight, masturbate your partner using your "wrong" hand. If you normally manually stimulate your partner with your right hand, then use your left hand this time. Hold your hands in front of you as if they are wrapped around the shaft of a penis. As you can see, by changing hands, you change which side of the penis is in your palm and which side is under your fingertips. This seemingly minor change significantly alters the sensations!

Use long, slow strokes that rub the penis from the base to the head. Steadily shorten the stroke and increase the pace. Go back to long, slow strokes. This is such a tease, but guys love it! Again, shorten the stroke and accelerate the speed. This time, continue the short strokes until your partner climaxes.

Knock Her Socks Off

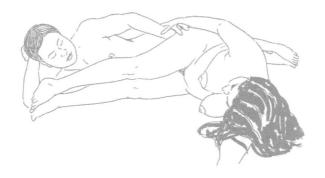

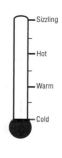

Sizzling

Hot

Warm

Cold

Socks and sex do not mix! So, guys, take her socks off and then knock her socks off!

This is an interesting position where both the man and woman are lying on their sides. The man is lying completely straight. The woman is bent at the hips so that her upper body is perpendicular to the man's body and her legs are against the man's chest. It looks a lot like a position where the woman is sitting on top of the man, except that they've tipped over onto their sides! The easiest way to achieve penetration is for the man to hold his penis steady while the woman moves her hips close to her partner.

Guys, as your partner moves closer to you, guide her hips so that the tip of your penis lines up directly with her vagina. You'll achieve full penetration once your partner's bottom is against your torso and her legs are against your chest. As a result, you've also got her feet right by your face. For many women, the feet are an erogenous zone. Massage them. Tickle them. Suck on her toes. If your partner is one of these women, she'll love all of this! It's guaranteed to knock her socks off!

Skin and Boners

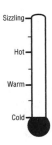

Sizzling
Hot
Warm
Cold

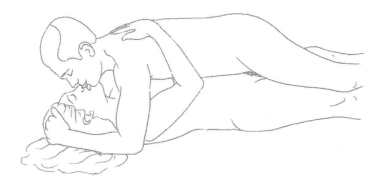

This position gives you both! Especially, lots and lots of skin contact! For best results, put a little oil or lotion on your skin before starting.

Guys, have your partner lie on her back. Lie down on top of her. Use your arms to take some of your weight off your partner. She'll appreciate this! Believe me, it's hard to fully enjoy a position when your lungs are about to collapse!

You and your partner should both have your legs spread open. Rest your thighs on her thighs. Hook your leg under her foot.

Have as much of your skin touching your partner's skin as possible.

Thrust your boner in and out. Slide your skin against her skin. Enjoy a very pleasurable and intimate position!

Standing Room Only

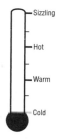

Sizzling

Hot

Warm

Cold

Shower stall, pantry, airplane bathroom, supply closet at work: What do all these places have in common? They're all perfect locations for the Standing Room Only position!

The trickiest part of this position is establishing penetration. Guys, bend your knees and lower your hips so that your penis is below your partner's vagina. Insert the tip and then straighten your legs to get fully penetrated. Ladies, start out on your tiptoes. This will elevate your vagina, making it much easier for your partner to reach it. Once your lover has inserted the head of the penis, lower yourself back down.

Guys, put your arms around your partner. Fondle and caress her breasts while she manually stimulates her clitoris. Penetration with this position is not particularly deep, but it is very tight. Try to hold off on your orgasm until you feel your partner's vaginal muscles tighten around your penis while she climaxes.

This is a standard rear-entry position that has probably existed forever. And as long as there continues to be small bathrooms and irresistible urges for a quickie, it will continue to exist!

Reflections

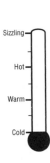

Sizzling

Hot

Warm

Cold

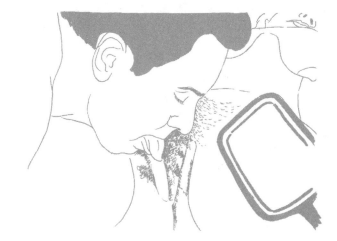

It's no secret that men are very visually stimulated. Just remembering the image of their penis sliding in and out of their partner's mouth is enough to give most guys a hard-on. With the help of a mirror, this cunnilingus activity gives women a chance to see some erotica of their own!

Ladies, get a mirror and get comfortable. Position the mirror so that you can see your entire vulva. You'll need to make adjustments as your partner moves around. Enjoy the physical and visual sensations as your partner performs cunnilingus.

Guys, give her a show she'll never forget. The secret is to show lots of tongue, so don't latch your mouth around her clitoris until you're ready for her to orgasm.

Stick your tongue out and very deliberately lick the whole area around her clitoris. Use your tongue to spread apart her labia and lick from her clitoris down to her vagina. Point your tongue and let her watch you dart it into and out of her vagina. Seeing your tongue disappear inside of her is intensely stimulating! Slowly lick your way back up to her clitoris. Flatten your tongue and lick back and forth over her clitoris. Bring her to orgasm by sealing your mouth around the clitoral area and rubbing the clitoris with your tongue.

This is an activity she is not going to forget. When you see her smiling to herself while making dinner, driving in the car, or drying her hair, you'll know what she's thinking about!

Choosing Sides

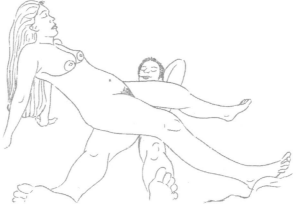

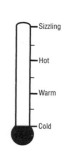

Sometimes, choosing sides can be so difficult. But not this time! Whether you choose to face his right side or his left side, this position feels great!

Ladies, have your partner lie on his back. Sit on top of your partner facing to the side. Use your hand to help guide his penis while you lower your hips. It's important that the head of the penis is over your pelvic bone before you attempt full penetration. Spread your legs wide open in front of you. Put your arms behind you and lean backward.

Guys, reach over and put your hand between your partner's legs. Feel her push against your hand each time she thrusts. Use the heel of your hand to stimulate her clitoris while holding the base of your penis with your fingers. Feel how hot and wet she is as she climaxes!

Left or right? For once, there are no wrong answers!

Whipped Cream and Nuts

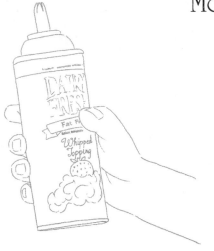

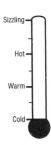

Sizzling

Hot

Warm

Cold

Get out the can of whipped cream, ladies! This is a food and fellatio activity! Start with the toes and start working your way up. I think you can pretty much figure out where we'll be going.

Spray whipped cream on and between your partner's toes. Put as many of his toes into your mouth as you can. The combination of the cold whipped cream and your hot mouth is very erotic! Suck the whipped cream off the toes one by one.

Spray whipped cream up the inside of his leg, particularly the top of his thigh. Flatten your tongue and lick your way from his ankles to his groin. Let your tongue tease and tickle all the way up.

Apply a dollop of whipped cream onto the tip of his penis. Take the complete penis head into your mouth and suck off the whipped cream. Again, the cold whipped cream and your hot mouth make an

overwhelming combination of sensations! Liberally coat his entire penis and testicles with whipped cream. Continue licking and sucking it clean until your partner has added some cream of his own.

Oh, and the next time you order dessert with whipped cream, ceremoniously use your tongue to lick some of it from your spoon. Trust me, he'll remember!

Back in the Saddle Again

Month 5

Day 28

Sizzling

Hot

Warm

Cold

Giddy-up cowgirls! It's time to go horseback riding!

Ladies, lasso your partner. Have him lie on his back with his legs bent at the knees. You'll be on top facing toward his head. Be sure to insert his saddle horn when you mount him! Spread your legs apart wide in front of you.

Start the horse at a slow pace. Rock your hips back and forth in the saddle as your horse moves up and down. Give your horse a little slap to the back leg, and increase the speed to an easy canter. You're still far away from your destination, and you don't want your horse to tire too

soon! As you see the end of your trip in sight, let the horse gallop at full speed. It's perfectly normal for him to froth and foam a bit from the exertion. Towel him down once the ride is over.

Tell your partner what a great stud he is and promise to visit his stable again soon!

Neck and Neck

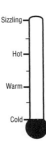

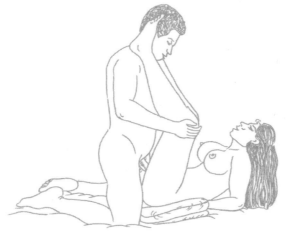

For this position, the woman lies on her back. Ladies, bend your arms behind you and rest your weight on your elbows. This will elevate your shoulders and head. Start with your legs bent and spread wide open. Put a pillow or two under your hips to make penetration easier.

Guys, kneel down between the woman's legs. Lift up her legs so her feet are on your shoulders. Lean against them to help you keep your balance. Place your hands under her hips, insert the head of your penis into her vagina, and then thrust your hips forward for full penetration.

Rub your hands along her calves and thighs while you thrust. Kiss her ankles and her toes. Tickle the bottom of her foot with your tongue. Pull your lover's hips to you as you experience the deep and satisfying orgasm.

Bottom Feeder

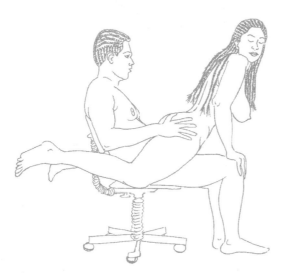

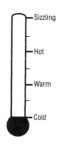

Sizzling

Hot

Warm

Cold

Guys who like bottoms will love this position!

Ladies, have your partner sit comfortably in a chair. Straddle his lap so that you are facing outward. Put your hands on your partner's knees and lean forward, putting your weight on your arms. Stretch your legs out behind you. Have your partner maneuver your hips so that you can move yourself backward onto his penis. Lift and lower your bottom up and down the shaft of his penis.

Guys, this is a great position for a little bottom action! Knead your fingers through the soft fleshy cheeks. Spank her. Many women find the sharp stinging of a good spank to be very stimulating. Separate her cheeks and tickle her anus. Encourage your lover to let you use some lubrication and try some anal penetration with your finger. The intensity will amaze her!

6 MONTH 6

Day 1. G That Spot
Feels Good

Day 2. Right Angles Can't
Be Wrong

Day 3. Hung Out to Dry

Day 4. Heads Up

Day 5. Flagpole Sitting

Day 6. Breath of Fresh Air

Day 7. Trusty Mechanic

Day 8. Shoulder Pads

Day 9. Tail Wagging the Dog

Day 10. Hit the Nail on the
Head

Day 11. Standing Your Ground

Day 12. Table for Two Please

Day 13. Uninterrupted Power
Supply

Day 14. Forbidden Fruit

Day 15. Carbon Copy

Day 16. Taking It Off and
Getting It On

Day 17. Silkworm

Day 18. All Systems Go

Day 19. Couch Potato

Day 20. Sidetracked

Day 21. Four-Course Meal

Day 22. Ring Around the
Collar

Day 23. Wet Your Whistle

Day 24. Fantasy Island

Day 25. Giving Her the Finger

Day 26. Take Me Out to
the Ball Game

Day 27. You'd Have to Be
Crazy

Day 28. Have It Your Way

Day 29. Sticks and Stones

Day 30. Dancing in the Sheets

G That Spot Feels Good

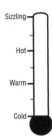

Sizzling

Hot

Warm

Cold

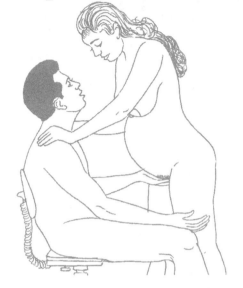

And, this spot feels really good!

Guys, this is a position where you manually stimulate your partner. Sit comfortably in a chair with your partner standing in front of you. Her legs should be spread wide open. Let her lean forward against your shoulders for balance.

Your job is to find your lover's G-spot. Don't panic! If you've never tried this before, it might seem a little daunting. But it's not that

hard! Read the instructions and give it a try.

The G-spot can be found on the front wall of the vagina. It's a dime-sized rough spot that is typically about two inches from the entrance of the vagina. Of course, all this varies from woman to woman. That's why this can be so challenging! Your lover's G-spot could be slightly bigger or smaller. It could be deeper inside or closer to the front of the vagina.

Insert your finger into your lover's vagina. Rub it along the front wall trying to find a small ridged spot. Press down on the spot. If it makes your lover feel as if she needs to use the bathroom, then it's probably her G-spot. Firmly rub your fingers against it while simultaneously using your other hand to masturbate her clitoris. Her orgasm will be very deep and intense!

Right Angles Can't Be Wrong

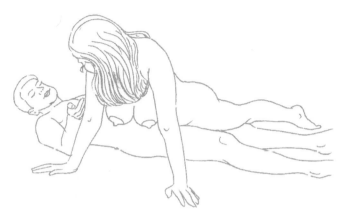

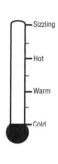

- Sizzling
- Hot
- Warm
- Cold

The right angles made in this position definitely feel right!

Ladies, have your partner lie flat on his back. Lie down sideways on top of him. Angle penetrations can be a bit tricky. Use your hand to guide his penis and tilt your hips to the side to help get started. Once his penis is snugly and warmly inside of you, rotate your hips so they are flat against your partner's hips, straighten your arms in front of you so that your weight is on your wrists, and open your legs wide behind you.

This is a great position for grinding your clitoris into your partner's hips. Move your hips around a bit until you find a spot on you that gets stimulated by a spot on him. Then, thrust your hips forward and backward, side to side, and around in a circle. Increase the pressure and pace until both of you climax.

Hung Out to Dry

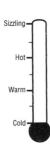

Sizzling
Hot
Warm
Cold

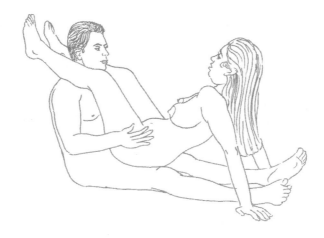

Her legs are hung over your shoulders, but it's anything but dry!

Guys, sit down on the bed with your legs straight in front of you. Have your partner sit down in your lap facing you. Slide your penis into her wonderfully wet vagina. As your partner leans backward onto her arms and hangs her legs on your shoulders, grasp her hips and pull her forward so that your entire penis is enclosed inside of her. Help her slide back and forth along the shaft of your penis. Clutch her hips to your pelvis and plunge as deeply as possible as you peak.

Ladies, give your partner some leg hugs. He loves to feel your soft silky skin up next to his face. Each time you tighten your legs around his head, tighten your vaginal muscles around his other head. The combination will drive him crazy!

Heads Up

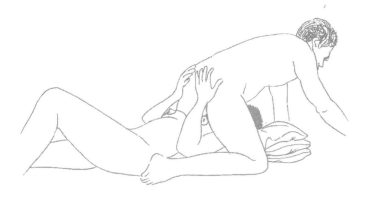

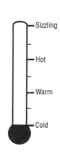

Sizzling

Hot

Warm

Cold

It's hot and wet. You love to slide in and out of it. It feels so good!

Okay guys, have you figured out yet which part of your partner we're describing? Let's add one more clue. It has a wickedly sweet tongue that can stimulate in ways that can't be paralleled anywhere else! Two body parts that are so similar, but so different.

This is a man-on-top fellatio position that allows for deep penetration and thrusting. Guys, have your partner lie on her back. Straddle her so that your legs are by her sides and your hands are over her head. Before you start thrusting, decide on a hand signal, like slapping your leg, that she can use when she needs you to pull out and give her a break. Nobody wants their obituary to read that they died of suffocation while giving a blow job.

Ladies, use your tongue! Let your partner slide in and out of your mouth as he thrusts his hips. Each time he pushes in, flick your tongue around on his penis. Sometimes focus on the head; sometimes focus on the shaft. Use a pointed tongue, a flat tongue, and vary the pressure. The intense stimulation will leave him begging for more!

Flagpole Sitting

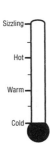

Sizzling

Hot

Warm

Cold

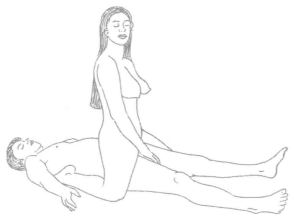

Flagpole sitting was a crazy fad that started in the 1920s. Supposedly, it died out by 1929. I'm not convinced!

Ladies, have your partner lie on his back with his legs spread wide open. Make sure his flagpole is fully erect. We're not interested in flying our flag at half-mast. Mount your partner, facing his feet. Your legs should be bent so that your feet are behind you.

Reach down between his legs and wrap your hand around his testicles. Hold them with your fingers while the heel of your hand stimulates your clitoris. Be careful not to squeeze too tight as your arousal increases. As you approach orgasm, move your fingers to the base of his penis. This slight movement provides a surge of excitement that will help you both climax at the same time.

Breath of Fresh Air

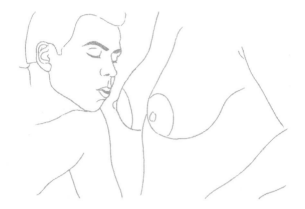

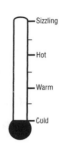

Sizzling

Hot

Warm

Cold

Your partner did this one for you, guys, now it's time to show her how good it feels. This is a cunnilingus activity where you wet your partner's skin and then blow on it. Start with the ears. Lick around the earlobes, and then softly blow on them. Although your breath is warm, it feels very tingly and cold when blown on the wet skin! Lick and blow on her neck, especially the spots you know are sensitive!

Work your way down to your partner's breasts. Flatten your tongue and lick the entire area around the nipple, making it nice and wet. Gently blow on the wet skin. It feels so cold and so arousing. Put your mouth around the entire nipple. The warmth of your mouth against the cold feeling of her skin is very stimulating. Pull your mouth back and blow directly on the nipple. This will send a shiver down her spine!

Gradually lick and blow your way from her breasts, across her tummy, to her clitoral area. Use your tongue to get her clitoral area wet. Very gently blow on her clitoris. For some women, this will cause some minor orgasms! Put your warm mouth around her cold clitoris and lick your tongue back and forth. After all this, she'll need a breath of fresh air.

Warning: Be careful not to get carried away with this activity. Blowing air on her clitoris is great. Blowing air into her vagina is not so great. A lot of women will find this extremely uncomfortable.

Trusty Mechanic

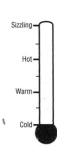

Sizzling

Hot

Warm

Cold

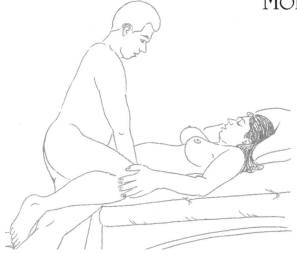

Time for a tune-up! And nobody can do it better than your trusty mechanic!

Guys, have your partner lie on her back with her legs hanging over the edge of the bed. Spread her legs apart so that they are opened wide. Kneel with one knee on the floor and one knee up on the bed.

The leg on the bed gives your engine some extra horsepower.

Insert your finger into your partner's engine. You need to verify that there's enough oil to keep all moving parts lubricated. Start your motor, letting the piston slide in and out of her engine.

Put your hands on your partner's breasts and massage them. This gives her battery a little extra juice. Continue shifting the engine into higher and higher gear until you have a blowout.

Whoever said car repairs are a hassle obviously doesn't have a mechanic like this!

Shoulder Pads

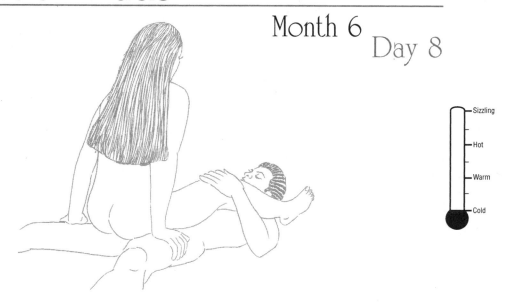

Sizzling

Hot

Warm

Cold

This is a very tight position that also gives the couple a chance to make great eye contact with each other. The man lies on his back with his legs spread open. The woman sits on top of the man with her legs as close together as possible without disrupting penetration. Her legs should be straight in front of her and on the man's shoulders.

Okay, guys, you've got your lover's legs right next to you. Use your hands to explore them and find some sensitive areas. If you've not tried this before, you might be surprised to find out that a woman's legs can be very erogenous. The trick is to find the right areas and learn how your partner likes to be touched. Try tickling your fingers along the outside of her thighs and calves. If she wants a less delicate touch, rub an area of skin back and forth or tap your fingertips against it. For some women, the sharp sensations of a light slap are very stimulating. Have your partner let you know when you've found a great spot. This activity is impossible without good feedback!

Watch your partner as she thrusts her hips up and down the shaft of your penis. Make eye contact with her as you tell her how much you love her. As you each approach your peaks, keep your hands on her legs, close your eyes, and just feel the sweet pleasure.

Tail Wagging the Dog

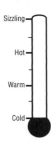

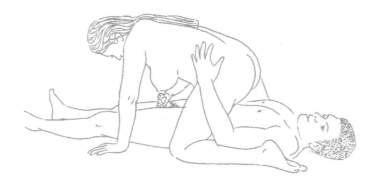

Okay, ladies. Time to manually stimulate your partner's bone. Have him lie flat on his back. Straddle your partner on your hands and knees so that your legs are up by his head and your hands are down by his other head.

Wrap your hand around the shaft of your lover's penis. Most people grasp the penis with their pinky finger near the base. This time, turn your hand around so that your index finger is near the base of the penis and your pinky finger is near the head. This slight change in the grip significantly alters the overall sensations!

Guys, enjoy the view as your lover straddles her bottom directly over your face. I'm sure she won't mind if you reach up and manually stimulate her. Or better yet, grasp her hips and lower her vulva to your face for some cunnilingus. A little tail is a great thing for this dog!

Hit the Nail on the Head

Month 6
Day 10

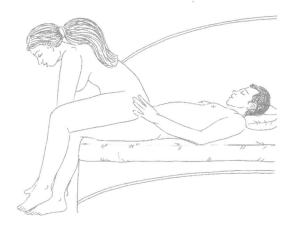

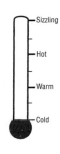

- Sizzling
- Hot
- Warm
- Cold

Ladies, you get to put the hammer down for this position! Have your partner lie on his back with his legs hanging over the edge of the bed. You will be sitting on his lap facing away from him. Place your hand around his nail to keep the head in place while you lower your hammer down his shaft. For the best results, be sure that the nail has completely penetrated. Place your legs on top of your partner's legs. This gives you maximum skin contact. Lean your upper body forward. This will ensure that the nail has a nice tight fit. Keep pounding your hammer up and down the shaft of his nail until both of you orgasm.

So, the age-old question "would you rather get hammered or nailed?" now has a whole new answer! He gets hammered while she gets nailed!

Standing Your Ground

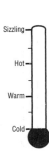

Sizzling

Hot

Warm

Cold

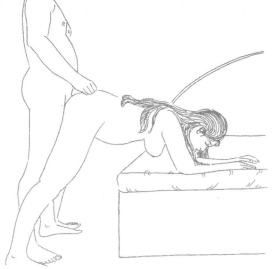

A rear-entry position with a bit of a different angle.

Guys, have your partner stand next to the bed and lean over so that her entire upper body is resting on the bed. Her legs should be spread open as wide as possible.

Stand behind your partner. Lift her hips to a height that allows penetration. It helps if she can be on her tiptoes and lift her bottom into the air. It also helps if you bend your knees a little. Lean into your lover as you slide your penis deep inside of her.

Ladies, while keeping your upper body resting against the bed, use one hand to reach down between your legs. Feel the base of your lover's penis as it slides in and out of you. It's erotic for you and very pleasurable for him!

Table for Two Please

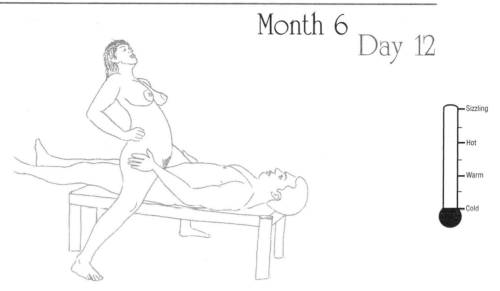

Sizzling

Hot

Warm

Cold

Preferably a quiet spot away from the windows!

This is a position where the woman's legs straddle the man (and the furniture) and reach down to the floor. So move the trusty coffee table to a good spot and get started!

Ladies, have your partner lie down on the coffee table with his legs out straight. Straddle your partner, facing him, but don't sit down yet. Grasp his penis with your hand and rub it all around your vulva. Let him feel how wet and hot you are for him. Insert the tip into your vagina and lower your bottom to his pelvis. Put your arms behind you and lean backward. Your partner will immediately notice how tight you've just become.

Guys, this is a position where you can enjoy the view. Watch your penis as it slides in and out of your lover. Reach over and manually stimulate her clitoris. Feel her vaginal muscles contract around your penis as she orgasms. Once she's reached her peak, continue thrusting until you've left a generous tip.

With service like this, you'll soon be regular customers at this table!

Uninterrupted Power Supply

Month 6
Day 13

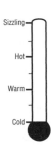

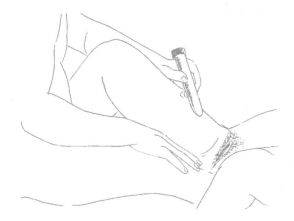

Check the batteries in the vibrator. There is nothing worse than running out of energy halfway through a great activity! You need an uninterrupted power supply for this one!

Guys, use the vibrator to manually stimulate your partner. Start by rubbing the vibrator against the bottoms of her feet. It tickles, but it feels great! Start moving the vibrator up her legs. Take your time. The calves, the backs of the knees, and the thighs can all be erogenous zones for some women. See if your partner is one of them.

When you get to the top of the thigh, shift over a bit and rub the vibrator around in her pubic hair. Spread your partner's legs open and move the vibrator to the clitoral area. Some women will experience small orgasms from this, but don't stop yet. Insert the vibrator into her vagina. Try and have the tip stimulate her G-spot on the front vaginal wall. Simultaneously, use your other hand to masturbate her clitoris. She's already very aroused from when you used the vibrator against her clitoris, so this should drive her wild. Bring her to a deep and powerful orgasm.

Forbidden Fruit

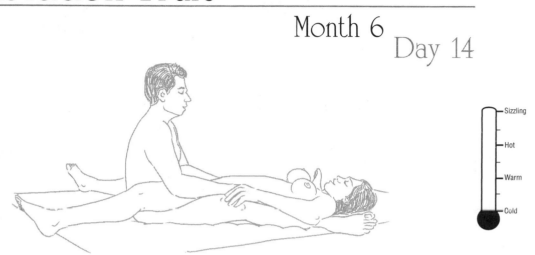

Sizzling

Hot

Warm

Cold

Orgasm is derived from the Greek word *orgasmos*, which means to grow ripe, swell, or be lustful. We can certainly do that with this position!

Ladies, have your partner sit on the bed with his legs spread open in front of him. Lower yourself to a sitting position on his lap facing him. Spread your legs out behind your partner as wide as you can so that all of his ripe fruit gets into your fruit basket. Lean backward until you are lying flat on your back.

Guys, do you see those golden delicious apples she has? Use your hands to polish and shine them. Move one hand to her clitoris for some manual stimulation. Feel her clitoris swell beneath your fingertips as her arousal ripens. Synchronize the thrusting of your hips and the movement of your fingers so that you can orgasm simultaneously.

Carbon Copy

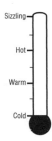

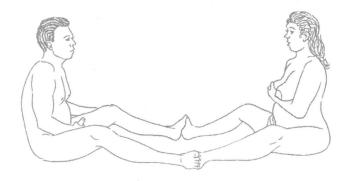

This is a position where each of you masturbates in front of the other. Sit facing each other with your legs spread open and your feet touching. If you prefer more skin contact, cross ankles with the woman's leg on top of the man's leg.

Decide who gets to go first. Some men can concentrate better on watching their partner when they are no longer concerned about taking care of themselves. Other men prefer to go second because once they orgasm, their interest in sex has decreased, making it more difficult to focus on their lover. Men that go second also find that the stimulation of seeing their partner go first improves their own arousal and masturbation. Decide what works best for you.

Watch your partner as they masturbate. Pay attention to how they use their hand, the amount of pressure they apply, and the tempo they use. Do they focus on a single area, like the head of the penis or the clitoris? Do they increase or decrease the speed as they approach their orgasm? Watch for minor details that will help you the next time you manually stimulate them.

Taking It Off and Getting It On!

Month 6
Day 16

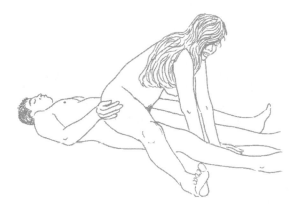

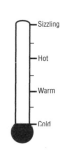

Okay, guys, time to do a little seductive striptease dancing for your lover. For those of you who have never done this or are a little nervous, relax! Women love to watch their lovers undress. You don't need great moves or an elaborate routine. Be creative and spontaneous. Have fun with it!

Once you've taken it all off, help your partner take her clothes off. Caress and kiss each body part as you uncover it. This is very romantic and very stimulating for both of you!

All right, ladies, now it's time to get it on. Have your partner lie on his back with his legs together straight in front of him. Climb on top of him facing his feet. Your legs should be spread open as wide as possible. After sliding your partner inside of you, lean forward. This will tighten your vagina and provide a lot more friction with each thrust.

Use your hands to rub his ankles, calves, knees, and thighs. Alternate between naughty and nice. Gently pull the hair or pinch the skin on his legs. Follow this with some delicate stroking that will tingle to his toes. As he approaches orgasm, focus more on naughty and less on nice. Just hold your hands against his legs as he reaches his peak.

Silkworm

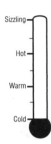

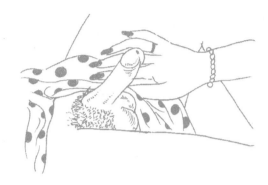

A silkworm is a larva that spins a silk cocoon. Ladies, this activity has you cocooning his worm in silk!

Find something silky that you can use for this activity. A silky nightgown or blouse works great. But make sure the item is washable.

Start by dragging the silk across his chest and stomach. The silk feels cool and sleek against your partner's skin. Drag it across his hips and pelvis. Each time the smooth silky fabric touches his worm, he will feel a rush of stimulation. Rub the silk against the head of his penis and then wrap it around the entire shaft. Use your hand to rub the silk up and down the shaft.

Because the fabric is so soft and slippery, use a full stroke, from base to head, to stimulate your lover. Use your other hand to hold his testicles inside a small silky cocoon of their own. Continue stroking the shaft until you bring your lover to a full orgasm.

All Systems Go

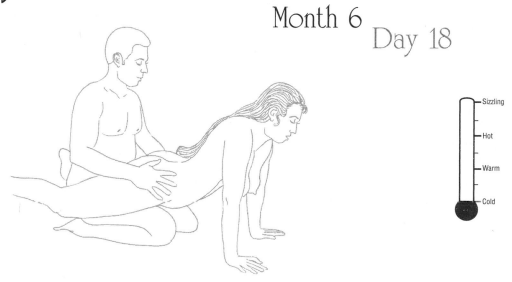

Sizzling

Hot

Warm

Cold

This position does not support remote dial-in access!

Ladies, have your partner kneel down on the floor with his legs completely bent underneath him. Do a quick hardware check. Be sure your partner has a good hard drive — a floppy just won't work! Put your hand on his joystick and lower yourself onto his laptop facing the same direction as your partner. Lean forward with your upper body resting on your arms. Stretch your legs out straight behind you.

Guys, put your hands all over the software that is in front of you. Grasp your partner's hips and pull her to you as close as possible.

This will give you the best connection for your cable and gives your partner's chip something to grind against! Massage her hips, buttocks, and lower back. Continue processing until all output has been printed.

Want to do it again? Just wait a few minutes and reboot the system!

Couch Potato

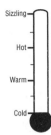

Sizzling

Hot

Warm

Cold

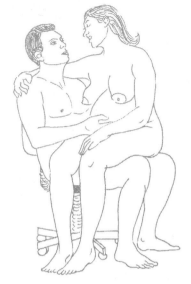

Any woman involved with a partner that likes to sit on the couch and watch TV is going to love this position!

Ladies, have your partner sit in a chair or on the couch and inform him that you will be controlling the remote. Lean over and kiss him seductively on the lips. Not too light and not too deep. Just enough to arouse his interest and make him want more. Bend over further and kiss his nipples. Feel them get hard under your lips.

Change the channel and lower yourself into his lap facing away from him. Use your hand to guide his antenna into your satellite dish. Carefully turn sideways so that both of your legs are on the same side of your partner's legs. This is a very tight position.

Guys, put your arms around your lover and hold her. Use your hands to massage her breasts. Pull gently on the nipples and rub them between your finger and thumb. It feels great and looks very arousing too. Hold your partner close and bury your face into her neck as you climax.

Check your local TV listings. I think this program is shown regularly!

Sidetracked

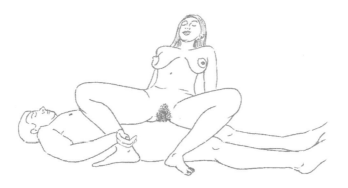

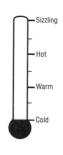

Sizzling

Hot

Warm

Cold

Turn off the TV and disconnect the phone. You don't want to get sidetracked while doing this position!

Ladies, have your partner lie flat on his back with his legs out straight. You'll be sitting sideways on top of him. You need your partner to be well lubricated for this position, so before climbing on board, lower your mouth onto his penis and get it nice and wet. Use your hand to insert the head of his penis into your vagina, and lower yourself down to your partner's hips. Remember that with sideways positions you need to be careful of your pelvis bone. The head of the penis must be inserted past the pelvis bone before full penetration will be possible. Spread your legs wide open and bend them so that your feet are sideways next to your partner's side. Put your arms behind you and lean backward.

Guys, use your hand to manually stimulate your partner. If you're really good, you can have one hand teasing her nipple while the other hand is stroking her clitoris. Not only will this intensify her orgasm, she'll be impressed too!

Four-Course Meal

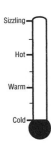

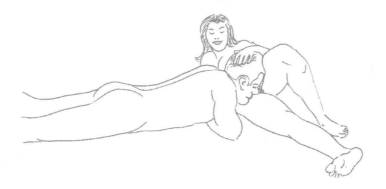

And, ladies, you are all four courses! So guys, get your mouth ready to do lots of eating!

Guys, have your partner lie on her side. You will be lying on your tummy perpendicular to your partner. Move around as necessary as you consume your way through the meal.

The first course is your partner's neck. Lightly rub your lips against the back of her neck. It will send a tickle down her spine! Lick and kiss her neck, working your way from her chin to her chest.

Course two is breasts. Hold your partner's breast in your hand and put your mouth around the entire areola. Use the tip of your tongue to lick back and forth across the nipple. Even when they are hard, wet nipples are so soft and pliable.

The vagina is course three. Lick the area around the vagina, and then move your tongue in and out. Point your tongue and lick the perineum. It's very sensitive!

The final course is, of course, the clitoris. Latch your mouth around the entire clitoral area, making it nice and wet. Use your tongue to rub back and forth over the clitoris. Feel it swell beneath your tongue as her arousal increases. Continue eating until she's had as many orgasms as she can handle!

Move over beef, chicken, and pasta. We've just found our new favorite meal.

Ring Around the Collar

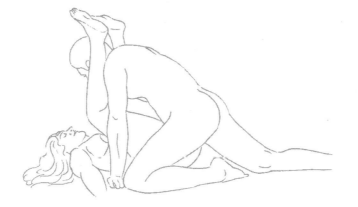

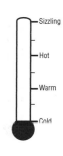

No scrubbing or soaking, and you definitely don't need any bleach! This is one ring around your collar that you want to keep!

Guys, have your partner lie on her back. Use your fingers to lightly rub against the opening of her vagina. Get your fingers wet and use them to lubricate the head of your penis. Use your hand to guide your penis and insert the tip into your partner's vagina. Lean forward for full penetration.

Move your arms one at a time so that your lover can lift her legs up to your shoulders. Feel how much deeper you can thrust now. Bend one of your legs and move the knee up next to your partner's bottom. This will change the angle of penetration and allow for stronger, deeper thrusting. Look your partner in the eye as you climax.

Wet Your Whistle

Sizzling

Hot

Warm

Cold

And then blow his whistle. This is a fellatio activity that requires your partner to be sitting in water. A hot tub, pool, or bathtub will work.

Take a deep breath and submerge your face into the water, putting your mouth around your partner's penis. The combination of the water around him and your mouth around his penis is incredibly stimulating for men. If the water is warm, like a bathtub or spa, your mouth will feel cold. Conversely, if the water is cold, like in a swimming pool, your mouth will feel very warm. Either way, men find this activity to be a huge turn-on.

This activity will rarely end in orgasm. It's just too difficult for the woman to keep her face underwater for that long. So after going down several times, switch to intercourse or manual stimulation. Your partner is already wet, slippery, and fully aroused. All he needs is a little help to push him to his peak.

Fantasy Island

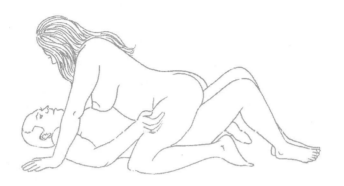

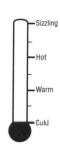

Fantasies. Everyone has them. Some, like performing fellatio on your partner at the movie theater, are achievable. Others, like having sex with your five favorite actors or actresses, are not.

Guys, lie down on your back with your legs bent at the knees. Have your partner straddle you with her legs bent so that her feet are behind her. Hold the shaft of your penis steady and let your lover lower herself down onto you. After penetration, your partner should lean all the way forward so that your heads are touching. Put your arms around her, hold her close, and tell her your secret fantasies.

Ladies, this is a chance to show what a great listener you are. Whatever fantasies your partner tells you about, don't be judgmental. These are fantasies and they belong to him. They don't reflect on you, and saying them out loud doesn't mean he plans to run off and act them out. However, if you hear some, like letting him shave off your pubic hair, that you are willing to try, let him know. It might be the best thing your sex life has seen since buying this book!

Giving Her the Finger

Month 6
Day 25

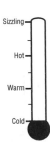

Sizzling

Hot

Warm

Cold

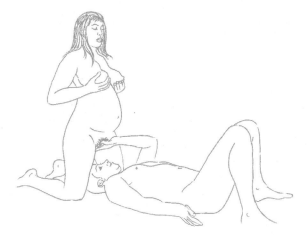

Guys, this is a position where you manually stimulate your partner. Your angle is a little different than usual, so if you've been having difficulty finding the spots that send her flying, this position might be the answer.

Lie on your back. Have your partner kneel by your head facing your body. Make sure her legs are spread apart. Reach your hand up behind you and stroke her inner thigh. Gradually move your hand over so that it's gently rubbing the labia and the area around her vagina. Try some soft pulls on her outer and inner lips. Some women are highly stimulated by this!

Rub your fingers in large circles around the entire clitoral area. Make the circles smaller and smaller until your fingers are nearly rubbing the clitoris directly.

Women can orgasm without direct clitoral stimulation. Continue rubbing circles around the clitoris. An indirect orgasm takes a little longer to develop, but it's worth the time and effort! Finish up with some direct clitoral stimulation. Continue rubbing your finger back and forth across her clitoris until she experiences a deep, satisfying orgasm.

Take Me Out to the Ball Game

Month 6
Day 26

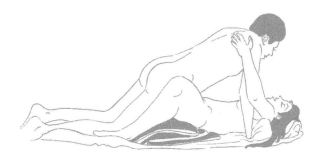

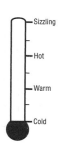

Play ball!

Guys, do you remember when you were younger and sexual conquests were described in terms of baseball? Kissing was getting to first. Getting your hand in her blouse was getting to second. Well, this position lets you run all the bases!

Get your bat ready because you're the next one up. Have your partner lie on her back. Put some pillows under her hips to elevate them. It makes penetration much easier. Her legs should be completely bent with her feet on their sides next to your legs.

Kneel down between your lover's legs. As you slide into home plate, lean forward so that your weight is on your arms. Kiss your partner's face and ears. Tell her what a great player she is and how glad you are to be on her team.

Take as many swings as you want. There are two balls and as many strikes as you need! So, keep the bat going until you've hit a home run!

Is the game over too soon? Why not make it a doubleheader?

You'd Have to Be Crazy

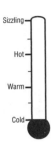

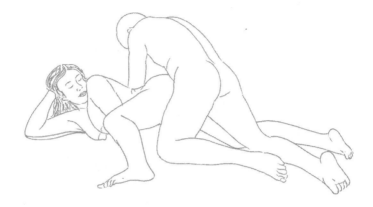

Not to like this one!
    The woman lies on her side. The man kneels facing the woman. The woman puts one of her legs between the man's legs. Her other leg is in front of her. If it's more comfortable, she can wrap her leg around her partner's waist.

    Penetration with this position is not very deep, but it is very tight. Ladies, clench your vaginal muscles each time your partner thrusts. It'll make things even tighter. Massage your breasts with your hands. Men are very visually stimulated and find it

pleasantly erotic to watch this. Seductively lick your finger and then rub it up against your nipple. If your partner wasn't crazy already, he'd have to be crazy now not to be enjoying this!

Have It Your Way

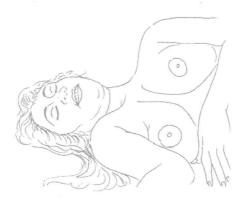

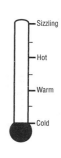

Ladies, for this intercourse activity, you get to have it your way. You get to choose the location, the foreplay, and the position. You get to tell your partner exactly what you want him to do.

For some of you, this will be very simple and a lot of fun! But for those of you who aren't used to saying what you want, this could be kind of challenging. Men really benefit when their partner clearly communicates her wants, needs, and desires. Do you want a little cunnilingus before intercourse? Tell him. Do you like to have your nipples sucked during intercourse? Tell him. Maybe you'd like him to use his finger and try some anal penetration during intercourse. Just let him know exactly what it is you want him to do.

So, you know what you want, but you're still not sure how you go about telling him. Well, assuming that neither of you only speaks a foreign language, I recommend plain, simple English. Talking about sex doesn't have to be vulgar or nasty, unless, of course, you want it to be. Keep things honest. Many women find it easier to talk about sex if they use anatomically correct terms, like vulva instead of pussy. Other women find just the opposite to be true. They would much rather call it his meat than say the word penis out loud.

One thing to remember as you go through this activity is that men really appreciate being told which things their partner particularly likes. This isn't an exercise in embarrassment. It's an attempt for honest, open communication that can greatly improve your sex life.

Sticks and Stones

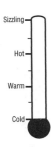

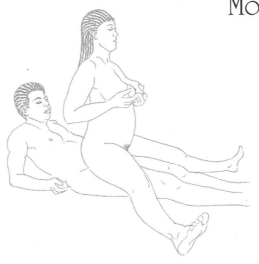

Have been known to break bones. But not with this position.

Ladies, have your partner lie on his back with his arms bent behind him and his upper body weight resting on his elbows. Facing the same direction, sit down on his hips with his stick in front of you between your legs. Rub your hands up, down, and all around the stick, making sure it's sturdy enough for the job. Move forward so that your pubic bone is right up against his stick. Clench your legs together, letting him feel how hot you are.

Lift up your bottom and use your hand to guide his stick inside your vagina. Lower your bottom back to his hips and spread your legs open as wide as possible. Reach down between your legs and put your hand around his stones. Polish them a bit with your fingers. Roll them around in the palm of your hand. Continue working the stick and feeling the stones until your partner orgasms.

Dancing in the Sheets

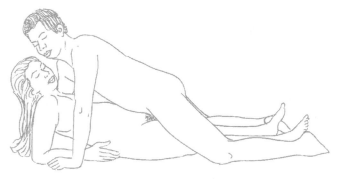

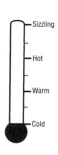

Sizzling

Hot

Warm

Cold

I suggest you make this a nice romantic slow dance. Dim the lights and put on some soft music. Start with lots of cuddling and kissing. Look at each other, touch each other, and truly enjoy being with your partner.

For this position, the woman lies on her back with her arms bent behind her to elevate her shoulders and chest. The man is in the basic missionary pose with his legs out behind him and his upper body weight resting on his arms in front of him. The woman should keep her legs as close together as possible. If it's comfortable, the woman can bend her legs and drape her ankles over the man's calves.

Notice how close you are to each other. Kiss the parts of your partner that you can reach. Talk quietly to each other. Remind your partner of their wonderful qualities that attracted you to them in the first place. After reaching your peak, thank your partner for the great sex.

MONTH 7

Day 1. Ice Princess

Day 2. Standing Ovation

Day 3. Don't Lose Your Head

Day 4. You've Got Mail

Day 5. Sit-down Strike

Day 6. Coming Around Full
Circle

Day 7. No Batteries Required

Day 8. Operators Standing By

Day 9. The Noose

Day 10. Mind Over Matter

Day 11. A Wing and a Prayer

Day 12. Double Your Pleasure

Day 13. War and Peace

Day 14. If the Shoe Fits . . .

Day 15. Fire Drill

Day 16. Looking Forward to This

Day 17. Dreaming of You

Day 18. Learning the Ropes

Day 19. The Poet

Day 20. Missionary Work

Day 21. Armchair Quarterback

Day 22. Twist and Shout

Day 23. Head of the Household

Day 24. Speak with a
Forked Tongue

Day 25. Sitting Duck

Day 26. Cat's Cradle

Day 27. The Pretzel

Day 28. Paying Lip Service

Day 29. Know When to Hold 'Em

Day 30. Getting Your
Wires Crossed

Ice Princess

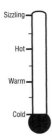

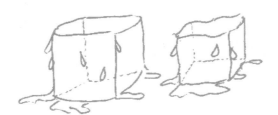

Okay, guys. Do you remember how much you enjoyed the Popsicle activity in month one? Well, this is your chance to let your partner experience the same wonderful sensations! So get a glass of ice and find a nice comfortable spot.

Start by using the ice on your partner's nipples. Get your mouth nice and cold and then surround her entire nipple with your chilly, wet mouth. If her nipples weren't erect already, they certainly will be now.

Gradually work your way down to her hottest parts. They definitely need to be cooled off! Take a small piece of ice and rub it all around the entrance to your lover's vagina. Don't let the ice cube stay in one spot for too long. We're not trying to inflict freezer burn. Push the ice cube into her vagina and move it around with your tongue. The combination of heat, wet, and cold is incredible!

Use another piece of ice to rub up and down the labia. These little flaps of skin sure do hold a lot of nerve endings! Get your mouth cold again and lower it onto her clitoris. Move your cold tongue back and forth and around in circles. Continue putting ice in your mouth to make it cold. Unless your partner agrees to it, never apply ice directly to her clitoris. For a lot of women, that is too much stimulation. For advanced stimulation, keep an ice cube in your mouth to prolong the cold spell.

Check the weather forecast for tomorrow. You might have to call in sick because of icy conditions.

Standing Ovation

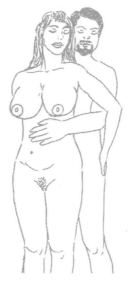

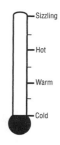

This is a very tight rear-entry position that will definitely have you cheering!

Both people are standing up for this one, facing the same direction. The woman (obviously) needs to be standing in front of the man. The trickiest part of this position is achieving penetration. Unless the woman is significantly taller than her partner, the man's penis is going to be pointing somewhere on her bottom or lower back. One option is for the woman to stand on something to make her taller. You don't need to add a lot of height, but she needs to stand on something wide enough for her to spread her feet apart. If you don't have something for the woman to stand on, then the woman should make herself taller by standing on her tiptoes while the man makes himself shorter by bending his knees. In either case, the woman should use her hand to guide the head of the penis to her vagina. For the tightest penetration, the woman should move her legs together until they are inside the man's legs.

Guys, put your arms around your partner and give her a tight squeeze. Nuzzle your nose up to her neck and ears. Keep one hand pressed right above her pubic hair. With a rear-entry position, this can accentuate the sensations she feels each time you thrust. It will also help hold her hips in place as your hips knock against her.

Standing ovations like this are usually followed by an encore. Guess you'll have to do it again!

Don't Lose Your Head

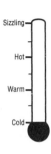

Sizzling

Hot

Warm

Cold

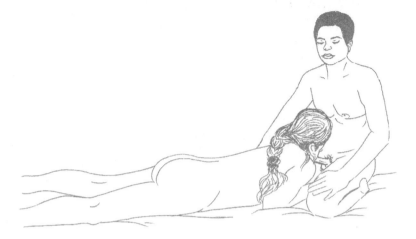

And for those women who don't like to swallow, don't let his head lose its load!

Ladies, lick your lips. This is a fellatio position and you want your lips to be smooth, soft, and wet! Have your partner kneel down with his legs completely bent so that his bottom is on the back of his calves. Spread your lover's knees apart and lie down on your tummy between them.

Start by kissing and sucking on his inner thigh. Unless he has a job that requires him to take off his pants, give him a nice hickey on the top of the inner thigh. It's a juvenile sign of ownership, and men love it!

Use your hand to grasp the shaft of his penis while you lower your mouth over the head. (If your mouth is a little dry, think about your favorite mouthwatering

dessert. This will help get your saliva flowing again.)

Move your hand and mouth simultaneously up and down the shaft and head of his penis. Let the tongue flick around each time the mouth is lowered. If you can, use your other hand to hold his testicles. Listen to him groan in pleasure as you slowly make him lose his head.

You've Got Mail

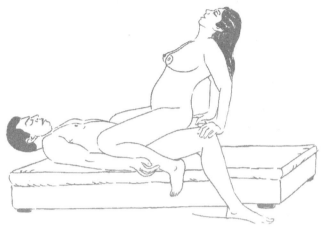

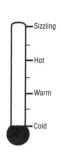

Sizzling

Hot

Warm

Cold

And the sweetest mailbox ever!

Ladies, surprise your partner with a secret message that is only for him. Prior to having sex, take a washable pen or marker and write a message to your partner on the very top of your inner thigh. Make sure you write it big enough that he'll be able to

see it. Your message can be romantic, seductive, or naughty. Whatever suits your personality—and his!

When you're ready for sex, have your partner straddle a bench or narrow table. His feet should be able to touch the ground. Sit on top of your partner facing his head. Your legs should be bent so that your

feet are behind you. Once you have him snugly inside of you, lean backward onto your arms and spread your knees apart. Watch your partner's face as he reads the message you've sent him!

He gets some mail and you get some male!

Sit-down Strike

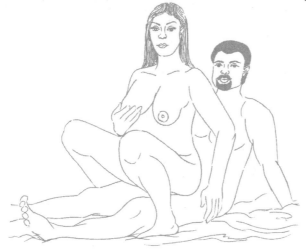

Sizzling

Hot

Warm

Cold

You don't have to join a union to participate in this sit-down strike. You can refuse to work, but there's no reason you should refuse to play!

Guys, sit down on the bed with your legs straight in front of you. Your partner will be sitting on top facing your feet. Her legs should be bent with her feet next to your thighs. Put your hands under your partner's bottom to help hold her up while she maneuvers her hips into position over the top of your penis. Feel the soft velvety warmth as your penis slides inside of her.

Ladies, spread your legs apart to allow for the deepest penetration. Put your hands between your legs. Let one hand hold your partner's testicles and use the other hand to masturbate. Pick an area that you want your partner to stimulate and let him know what it is. Maybe you like your nipples squeezed, your arms massaged, or your tummy stroked. Pick your pleasure. And tell your partner that you will be on strike until all your needs are completely satisfied!

Coming Around Full Circle

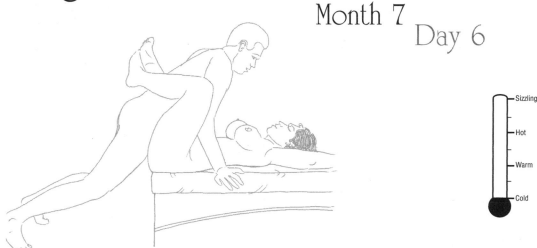

Sizzling

Hot

Warm

Cold

This is a very intimate and deep position!

Guys, have your partner lie on the bed with her bottom all the way to the edge and her legs hanging down the side. Spread her knees apart and stand between them. Bend over and use your tongue to make her nice and wet. Insert the head of your penis into her vagina. Lean forward with your arms in front of you on the bed. Extend your legs behind you and thrust your hips forward for full, hot penetration.

Ladies, once your partner has penetrated, lift your legs and wrap them around his waist. Tighten your legs and pull your lover's hips to you. He'll experience a sense of intimacy when he feels you pulling him closer to you.

He'll also feel a stimulating rush, as his thrusts can now be much deeper. For you, pulling him closer will allow your partner's hips to bump against your pelvis bone as he thrusts. Wiggle your hips around a bit until you find a sensitive spot that gets stimulated with each thrust. Clench your legs together as both of you reach your peaks.

No Batteries Required

Sizzling

Hot

Warm

Cold

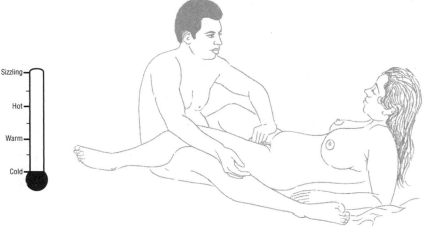

Guys, you supply all the energy that is needed by manually stimulating your partner in this position. Sit on the bed with your legs opened wide in front of you. Have your partner recline between your legs. Her legs should extend over your hips and straight behind you. Have her rest her weight on her elbows behind her. This allows for better eye contact as she watches you stimulate her.

Start by licking your fingers to get them lubricated. Then put one of the labia between your thumb and finger and gently rub back and forth. Use more lubrication as necessary until the labia are soft and wet.

Move from the outer lips to the inner lips using the same techniques. Massage the inner lips by rubbing them between your thumb and finger. Work your way

to the top of the lips and rub circles around the clitoris. Using either a circular or back-and-forth motion with your fingers, let your partner experience a wonderful orgasm.

As you try new things, encourage your partner to let you know what feels good. This is the only way you'll truly know the best ways to please her.

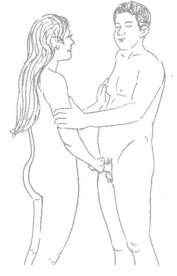

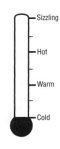

Sizzling

Hot

Warm

Cold

This position is great for the mornings when he's in need, but there isn't time for intercourse. Have your partner join you in the shower and manually stimulate him instead.

Ladies, have your partner stand in front of you. Stand close enough so that you can rub the head of his penis up against the smooth skin of your tummy. Wrap one hand around the shaft of his penis and start to stroke. Put the other hand over the head of his penis and rub it all over with your palm. Periodically, move the hand from the penis head to his testicles and hold them, rubbing his penis head against your tummy when you do this. Then, switch your hand back to the head of his penis again.

Guys, wrap your arms around your partner and hold her close. Snuggle your face into her neck. Be careful not to rest all of your weight on her. As you get more aroused, you'll start holding her tighter and leaning into her. Unless she has a wall behind her, you're going to eventually knock her off balance. Not exactly the ending either of you were counting on!

The Noose

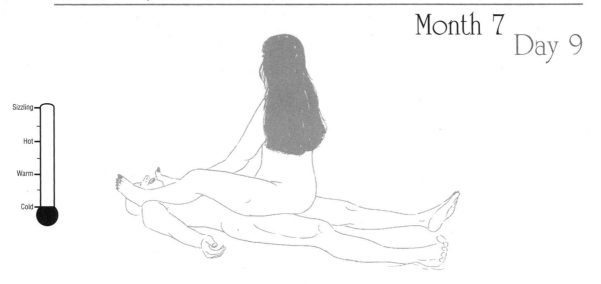

Sizzling—

Hot—

Warm—

Cold—

This position is for all you guys that think a serious relationship is a fate worse than death! Using this hangman's noose will definitely end your misery and increase your pleasure. That is, at least for a little while.

For this position, the guy lies on his back with his legs out straight. Ladies, face your partner and his hips, but keep his penis between your legs in front of you. Spread your legs open and use the head of his penis to stimulate your clitoris. This positively drives a man wild! Not only are the physical sensations intense, he also finds it incredibly arousing to watch. Continue rubbing yourself, switching to your fingers if necessary, until you orgasm.

Your partner can hardly wait another minute. He knows you're warm and wet and he definitely wants in. Raise your hips up over his penis, insert the tip into your vagina, and slowly slide down the shaft. Put your legs straight in front of you so that your feet are next to his neck. Every once in a while, squeeze your feet together so he can feel the noose tightening. Observe the intensity on his face as he orgasms.

Mind Over Matter

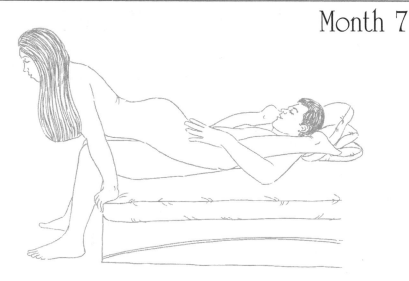

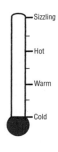

Sizzling

Hot

Warm

Cold

Ever have days where it seems like you have so much matter and so little mind? Well, for this position, you won't mind because it doesn't matter!

The man lies on his back with his legs over the edge of the bed. The woman is on top of the man, facing away from him. The easiest way to achieve penetration is for the woman to start out squatting over the man. Once she has him fully encased inside her, she can lean forward with her hands on her partner's thighs. Remember to do this slowly, because in most cases you will be bending the penis into an angle that is contrary to the way it normally hangs. While leaning forward, the woman should also stretch her legs out straight behind her.

Guys, this is a great position for using a lubricated vibrator to give your partner some anal penetration. If your partner has never tried this before, go slowly. She may seem a bit reluctant at first, but once she's tried it, chances are she'll love it! So, start by rubbing the vibrator up against her anus. Then, spread her cheeks apart and insert the vibrator inside of her. This is an incredibly powerful feeling! It won't cause her to orgasm, but she will feel a tingle from her scalp to her toes!

A Wing and a Prayer

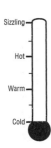

Sizzling

Hot

Warm

Cold

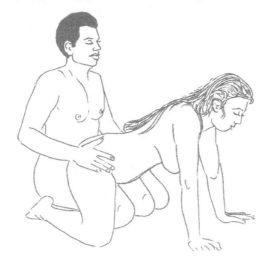

This expression originated during World War I when badly damaged aircraft would manage to land safely back at base. They were said to be flying on a wing and the prayers of the crew.

Guys, you get on your knees for this one, but I don't think you need to say any prayers for a happy ending. This position will have you both flying without any difficulties!

Ladies, after your partner is kneeling, climb on top so that you are both facing the same direction. Straddle his lap with your legs bent so that your feet are behind you. Once your partner is successfully inside of you, lean your upper body all the way forward. This will significantly tighten your vagina and increase the friction your partner feels when he thrusts. It'll also lift your bottom so that it's pressing up against your partner's tummy.

Guys, you have this beautiful woman in front of you and two free hands. Rub her shoulders, back, and sides. Use long strokes all the way from the bottom of her back to the top. Tap your fingers down her spine from her neck to her buttocks. Stroke, rub, pat, tickle, and massage while your thrusts take you both higher and higher. She'll love all of it!

Double Your Pleasure

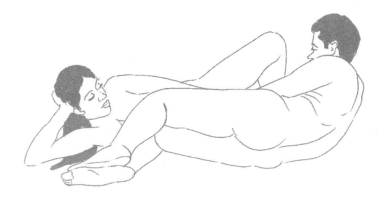

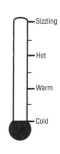

Sizzling

Hot

Warm

Cold

Have you ever tried to decide which is better — the physical pleasure you experience when your partner pleases you or the emotional and mental pleasure you experience when you please your partner? Well, with this position, you get to double your pleasure by having both! You will manually stimulate your partner and your partner will also be manually stimulating you.

Lie down in a reverse side-by-side position so that your heads are on opposite ends from each other. Start with some playful foreplay before getting to the serious stimulation. Look for some areas that haven't gotten any attention lately and tickle, stroke, or knead them. The idea here is to establish some physical, but not necessarily sexual, contact. Gradually increase the intensity and steadily

move toward stimulating the genitals.

It can be difficult to concentrate on both, but try to enjoy what you are doing as well as what is being done to you. As one of you approaches your peak, take a break from stimulating your partner, and thoroughly enjoy the physical sensations of being so well serviced!

War and Peace

Sizzling—

Hot—

Warm—

Cold—

Prepare for combat! We have a strategic initiative to implement, and the time to strike is right now.

Ladies, ambush your partner and have him lie on his back with his legs out straight. Reconnaissance photos have indicated that the best tactical maneuver is for you to sit on top facing your partner's feet. This is a naval assault, so be sure

you're very wet! Use your hand to help your partner's heat-seeking missile find its target. Once securely in place, spread your legs open wide, and rub your fingers against your clitoris. Continue stroking until you feel the explosive rush of climactic pleasure.

Guys, you are lying behind enemy lines. Escape can be found by using your

hands to help navigate the soft fields in front of you. Launch a rear assault by massaging, stroking, and tickling your partner's lower back and sides. The war is over once your missile has exploded.

Remember, all is fair in love and war. If once isn't enough, just declare war again.

If the Shoe Fits . . .

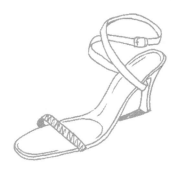

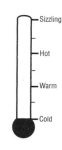

Wear it for this position!

Depending on your personality and wardrobe, this activity is either going to be very erotic and visually stimulating or playfully fun and lighthearted. Personally, I recommend the visually erotic. I think my husband would too.

If you want to try the sexy and erotic route, ladies, you need sexy and erotic shoes. Spiked heels work great. Little straps around the ankle are always a good turn-on. Leather boots up to the knees — awesome. Do some sensuous dancing and let your partner watch you strip down to your shoes. I think you can figure out what to do from there!

Okay, so you don't own any stripper shoes and you don't feel like buying or borrowing some for one activity. No problem! For the playfully fun version of this activity, any pair of shoes will work. Changing one dimension of your sexual environment can completely change the overall experience. Why do you think so many people have sex in unusual, and sometimes bizarre, locations? I don't think it was just to try a new position! For this activity, the aspect being changed is for both of you to keep your shoes on during intercourse. Your feet will be heavy and you'll probably feel a little silly. Have fun! Laughter and love are an enduring combination!

Fire Drill

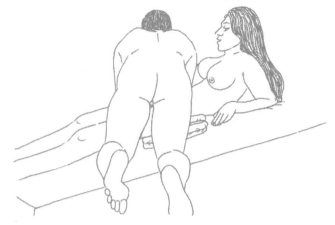

Sizzling

Hot

Warm

Cold

You have to start a fire before you can put out a fire. So, get things blazing with some scorching hot foreplay!

Get a deck of cards and get ready to play strip poker. Each time you win, you get to take an item of clothing off your partner. But you only get to use one hand. One hand removes the clothing, while the other hand arouses your partner by stroking,

rubbing, or massaging. Advanced players can try stripping their partners without using their hands at all. Of course, since the object of the game is to get naked, losing might actually be better than winning!

Once things are hot, call in the fire department. Guys, have your partner lie on her back with her arms bent behind her and her weight resting on her elbows. Kneel down next to

your partner and check for smoke. Rub your nose between her legs, using the tip to stimulate the area around her clitoris. Things are definitely hot! Lean your weight forward onto your arms, and insert your hose into her fire. Keep both of your partner's legs in front of you and position yourself so that you're at a 45 degree angle to her. Pump your hose until all flames have been extinguished.

Looking Forward to This

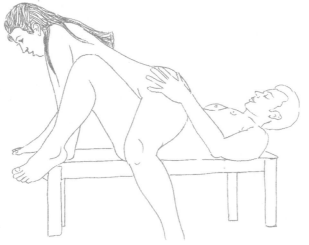

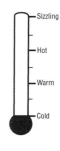

Anytime the woman sits backward and leans forward, the position is very tight! This position is no exception.

Use a bench, narrow table, or cot so that the woman can straddle her legs on either side. The man lies on his back on the table. His legs should be bent at the knees.

Ladies, you will be sitting on top of your partner facing his feet. Straddle your partner and scoot backward so that your vulva is over your partner's face. Ask him to make sure that you are very wet and then use your mouth to do the same for him. Move forward and let your partner's penis smoothly slide into your vagina while both of you are thoroughly lubricated.

Lean forward as far as you can between your partner's knees. Remember to take this slow — the penis can be broken! (It'll make a popping noise.) It usually occurs when the woman is on top! When done correctly, leaning forward will constrict the vagina, providing very tight penetration. Clench your vaginal muscles together to make things even tighter.

Hopefully you enjoyed this one and will look forward to leaning forward again soon.

Dreaming of You

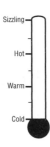

Sizzling

Hot

Warm

Cold

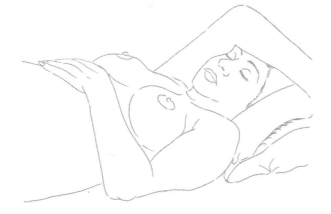

Hopefully, all you guys that tried this as a cunnilingus activity in Month 1 were successful. If not, here's your chance to try and stimulate your partner in her sleep again. This time the task is to manually stimulate her with your hand. Most guys seem to find this activity a little bit easier.

If you're extremely lucky, your partner is lying on her back with her legs spread apart. This might happen to about one in a thousand of you! The rest of you will have to be more industrious with your approach. The goal is to get your hand between her legs and stimulate her. In most cases, you won't have enough room to move your hand sufficiently to cause her to orgasm. What should happen, however, is that you can arouse her to a level so that when she wakes up she will already be hot and wet.

Once she's awake, you can either continue stimulating her by hand, or you can decide together that you'd rather have intercourse. Either way, her dream is not complete until you've brought her to her peak.

Learning the Ropes

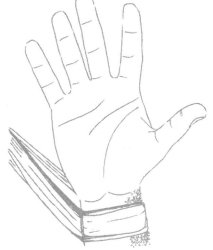

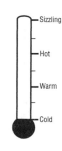

Sizzling

Hot

Warm

Cold

Time to get some nylons, rope, or soft scarves. The ladies get to tie up the men and then manually stimulate them. Guys that always like to be in control might have a hard time adjusting to this activity. The rest of the guys (most of you, in fact) will immediately love it!

Tie up your partner's hands either to each other or to the bed. You can optionally tie his ankles to the bed too. Your goal is to tease and arouse him until he's begging you to make him come. Rub your fingers against his nipples, making them taut. Kiss them, lick them, suck them, gently bite them. Pull away and move down his tummy to his groin. Use your hand and give him a few strokes along his shaft. Tell him it feels a little dry and then lower your mouth over his penis and get it fully lubricated. Give him a few more strokes. Wrap your hand around his testicles and roll them around. Again, give him a few strokes. Rub the head of his penis against the palm of your hand and then give him some more strokes. Continue alternating between a nonstroking activity and stroking until he can't stand it any longer. Fully stroke the shaft and head of your partner's penis until he orgasms.

The Poet

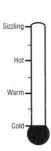

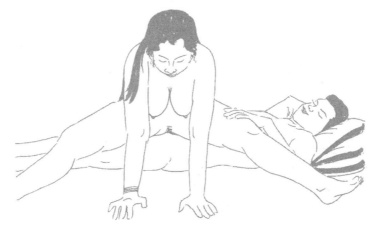

The man is on his back
  His penis standing straight
His partner's hot and wet
  It's time to penetrate.

The woman sits on top
  With her legs spread open wide
Not facing forward or backward
  Her legs are to the side.

The woman should lean forward
  This makes everything so tight
Penetration at this angle
  Feels so superbly right!

Rub your hips into his pelvis
  It feels so good to grind
Try all sorts of new maneuvers
  Guaranteed to blow his mind.

You need some stimulation
  Put your hand upon your clit
Rub it back and forth
  Feel the fire that's been lit.

Sex is so dynamic
  It's satisfaction that you seek
Keep the action going
  Till you both have reached your peak.

Missionary Work

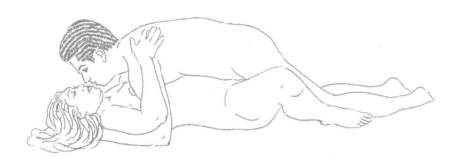

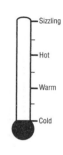

Sizzling

Hot

Warm

Cold

What comes to mind when you think of missionary work? The hot jungles of Africa? The selfless sacrifice and hard work? How about the sexual position? For most of us, this is as close to missionary work as we'll ever get. And this missionary work is really play!

This position is a variation of the standard missionary position. Like the standard position, the woman is lying on her back. The man spreads her legs and penetrates her in the standard missionary pose with his arms in front of him and his legs straight behind him. Unlike the standard missionary position, the woman should have one leg completely bent so that her foot is by the man's hip. Her other leg should be wrapped around her partner's waist.

Tonight, before having sex, change the light bulb in your lamp to a colored bulb. Red, green, blue, purple, orange. The color doesn't matter as long as it's not a standard white bulb. The entire ambience of the room will change. It becomes more romantic, but also more electric. Bodies and faces look different. Since we are so visually stimulated, when things look different, we actually think they feel different!

Colored light and the unusual position of the woman's legs make everything seem fresh and different again. Try experimenting with different colors to see if they provoke different moods.

Armchair Quarterback

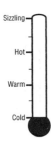

Sizzling

Hot

Warm

Cold

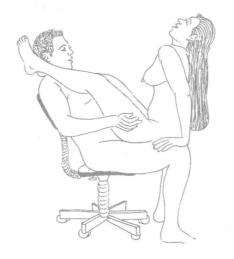

It's first and ten. Get into the huddle with your partner and work out the play. We don't want a false start or pass interference tonight!

Guys, sit down comfortably in a chair. This play requires your partner to sit in your lap. Insert your penis into her vagina as she lowers herself down into your lap. This play does not involve the tight end. Attempt to include this player and your partner will penalize you for being offsides.

Once penetration is complete, and there are no flags on the play, have your partner lean backward and put her legs up around your neck. You definitely want to help her with this. Reach out and massage your partner's breasts. No infraction of the rules for holding these! Continue making plays until you've scored a touchdown.

And just something to keep in mind. You get lots of extra points for helping your partner score. This is one time the quarterback won't mind being sacked!

Twist and Shout

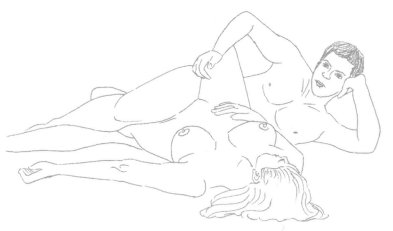

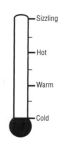

Sizzling

Hot

Warm

Cold

Come on, come on, come on, baby now.

For this twisted position, the man lies on his side. The woman lies on her back perpendicular to her partner. She has one leg entwined between her partner's legs and one leg bent over his hips. Her hips will need to be twisted to the side a little bit to allow penetration.

This position is not very deep, but it is very stimulating for the woman. Guys, your thigh is resting right on her pubic bone. Encourage your partner to slide her hips around until a sensitive spot is pressed up against you. Then, press down with your leg each time you thrust. Watch as her hips rise up to meet your leg as she gets more and more aroused. Feel her vaginal muscles contract as she orgasms, and gives a great shout.

Head of the Household

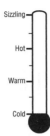

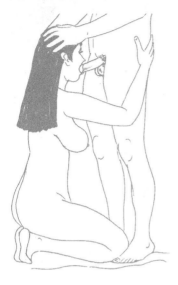

So, who wears the pants in your household? Well, when you're offering to give him head, I suspect he'll have no problem agreeing that you should wear the pants instead of him!

This is a very classic oral sex position with the man standing and the woman kneeling at his feet. Some men like to lean backward with a wall behind them to hold some of their weight. Others prefer to have a wall in front of them so that they can lean forward. And, of course, there are always those with enough balance that they don't need to lean against anything, even when someone is performing fellatio for them while they stand.

Ladies, get on your knees in front of your partner. With one hand wrapped around the shaft and your other hand holding his testicles, lower your mouth over the head of your partner's penis. Use your tongue to lick around the outside edge. Run your tongue up and down the slit in the back. Flatten your tongue and rub it all around the head's surface.

Despite the myths, there is no need to try and deep-throat his entire penis. The head is the most sensitive part. Doesn't it make sense that this should be the portion stimulated by your tongue? Use your hand to stroke his shaft while your tongue is exploring, licking, rubbing, and stimulating the head. He'll have no trouble reaching his peak.

Speak with a Forked Tongue

Month 7
Day 24

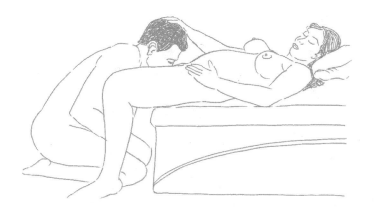

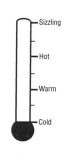

Sizzling

Hot

Warm

Cold

Can you imagine how great cunnilingus would be if a guy's tongue was forked and had two tips moving around independently of each other? Not to say that their tongues aren't pretty good already. But, two tips? Thankfully, it doesn't cost anything to dream!

Guys, have your partner lie on her back with her legs hanging over the edge of the bed. Spread her legs open nice and wide. Start by leaning forward to kiss and lick her breasts. Stick your tongue out all the way and let your lover watch you licking her nipple. Women are visually stimulated too!

Get your tongue extra wet and drag it from her breasts down her tummy to her pubic hair. Use your fingers to spread apart her labia. Then, lower your mouth to her clitoral area. Let your nose rub against her pelvic bone while your tongue is working around the clitoris. This will almost make it feel as if you've got two tongues! To totally put her over the top, use your finger to stimulate the outside of her anus, particularly the very sensitive perineum. Let her rock her hips as you bring her to her climax.

She won't be speaking with a forked tongue when she tells you how much she loved it!

Sitting Duck

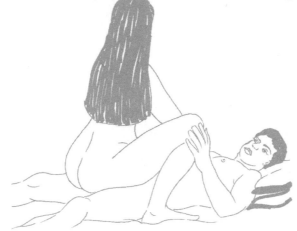

Sizzling

Hot

Warm

Cold

Time for target practice. And a sitting duck is one of the easiest targets that exist!

Guys, lie on your back with your legs spread open wide. Your partner will be the sitting duck on top of you. Have your partner facing you with her legs bent so that her feet are flat on the bed next to your hips. A moving target is hard to hit, so hold your partner's hips steady while you shoot your arrow inside of her. Long, straight, and deep. Another bull's-eye. You must be an expert archer!

Now, guys, you can earn some bonus points while you're thrusting. Use your hand to try to find the more difficult target — the spot on your partner that gives her an intense orgasm. Start by closing your partner's inner and outer lips. You'll get to open these back up like presents as you stimulate her. First use several fingers to stimulate the area with the skin closed. It's not intense for your partner, but it's still very pleasant. Then, open the outer lips, keeping the

inner lips still closed. Stroke them and rub them between your fingers.

With two fingers, spread the inner lips apart. Her inner lips form her clitoris hood, so when you spread them apart her clitoris will be visible. Rub your fingers in circles around the clitoris. If your partner is highly sensitive, fold the inner lips back over the clitoris and stimulate her through the skin. Either way, she'll think you're an excellent marksman as you bring her to orgasm.

Cat's Cradle

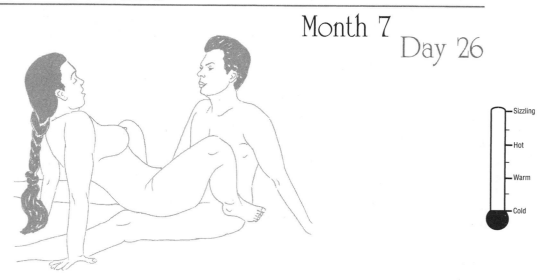

Sizzling

Hot

Warm

Cold

We're not talking about a child's string game. Rock this pussycat's cradle, but don't plan on sleeping!

Ladies, after your partner is sitting on the floor with his legs spread open in front of him, lower your pussycat down onto his scratching post. Bend your legs over your partner's thighs so that your feet are by his hips. Lean backward with your arms behind you.

Guys, use your hand to rock her cat's cradle. Stroke her fur while rubbing her clitoris back and forth. Her purring will let you know when you've found a good spot. After your partner orgasms, put your hands under her hips to help them rock back and forth. Continue rocking her cradle until you climax.

The Pretzel

Sizzling

Hot

Warm

Cold

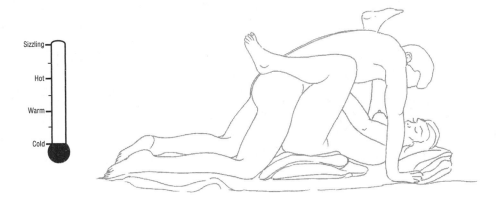

Open a cold frosty one while doing this position. Pretzels always taste best with beer!

For this position, the woman lies on her back. To help penetration, she should use a pillow or two to elevate her hips. The man kneels between the woman's legs and leans forward with his weight resting on his arms. One of the woman's legs should be up by her partner's neck. Her other leg should be wrapped around his waist.

Guys, there are a few things you can do to increase the intimacy of this position even more. Start by smiling at your partner. Let her know you're happy to be there with her. Make eye contact with your partner. Call your partner by her first name, not sweetheart or some nickname. Women love being called by name during sex! It really makes them feel so close to their partner.

A word of caution: If you have a lot of partners or have just started dating the woman you're with, be careful to use the right name. Nothing will end great sex quicker than using another woman's name in bed!

Ladies, pull your partner to you with the leg that you have wrapped around his waist. Men loved to be squeezed into a leg lock! This will also increase your chance for an orgasm as he bumps up against your pelvic bone each time he thrusts.

Thankfully, pretzels are low in fat. You can indulge again and again and again.

Paying Lip Service

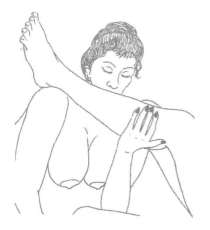

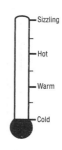

Sizzling

Hot

Warm

Cold

Ladies, you'll be paying lip service to all three of your partner's legs during this fellatio activity. Use your tongue and lips to fully explore your partner's legs, looking for new sensitive areas. Start with the ankle. This bony part of the anatomy is frequently overlooked, but can be sensitive and erogenous, especially when tickled by the tongue. Slowly work your way up your partner's calves and thighs. Kiss, lick, suck, and bite. Make sure your partner gives you some feedback so you'll know which spots need a return visit in the future.

As you approach the top of your partner's leg, focus on the areas around his penis. Lift his penis up with your hand and kiss and lick the skin on his torso underneath it. Let the head of his penis rub against your face and hair while you do this. With just your lips (no tongue), kiss the tip of your partner's penis. Follow this with small kisses all around the head and shaft. You know he wants more, but make him wait. Add a bit of tongue to your kisses, gradually increasing the amount of licking and decreasing the amount of kissing. Finally, use your whole mouth and give him what he wants. Close your mouth around the head of his penis. Lift and lower your head around his shaft until he reaches his peak.

Know When to Hold 'Em

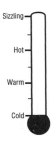

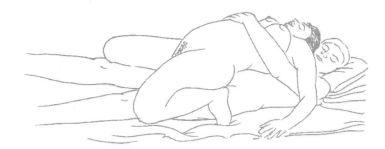

And know when to fold 'em. Guys, with this intimate position you can do both as you fold your arms around your lover and hold her tight.

Start by lying down on your back with your legs spread apart. This will give your legs some leverage for thrusting. Have your partner sit on top of you facing your feet. Her legs should be bent so that her feet are behind her. Put your hands on her hips to help maneuver her onto your penis.

Help your partner as she lowers herself backward down onto your chest. Feel her vagina lengthen as she brings herself down. Put your arms around your partner and hold her close. Kiss her neck and ears. Whisper in her ear how good it feels to be so deep inside of her. Encourage your partner to masturbate and enjoy the sensation as her hips grind into yours. Hold still and enjoy each other even after both of you have peaked.

Getting Your Wires Crossed

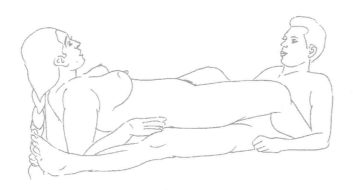

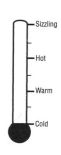

It's okay to get your wires crossed with this high-voltage position. We want lots of electricity to be flowing.

For this position, the man is reclining on his back with his arms bent behind him and his weight on his elbows.

Ladies, sit down on your partner's lap facing him.

Using your hand, guide your partner's wire into your circuit board and feel the electricity start flowing. Lean backward, putting your weight on your arms behind you. This will tighten your vagina and prevent any loose connections. Wrap your legs around your partner's waist.

Move your hips forward and backward to generate an electrical current.

Guys, reach forward and use your hand to generate some friction around your partner's clitoris. Continue conducting electricity until you've overloaded the system and both of you have blown a fuse!

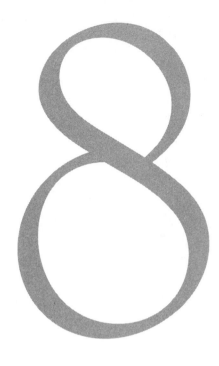

MONTH 8

Day 1. A Bone to Pick with You

Day 2. Bench Presses

Day 3. In Your Face

Day 4. Shop Till You Pop

Day 5. Complimentary Angles

Day 6. Touch of Class

Day 7. Winner's Circle

Day 8. Cream of the Crop

Day 9. One-Night Stand

Day 10. Down and Dirty

Day 11. The Corkscrew

Day 12. Every Dog Has
His Day

Day 13. Dancing on Tables

Day 14. Face the Music

Day 15. Best Seat in the
House

Day 16. Mixed Nuts

Day 17. Honey, We're Eating
Out Tonight

Day 18. Knock on Woody

Day 19. Sitting Pretty

Day 20. Growing Season

Day 21. Full-Court Press

Day 22. Tongue in Cheek

Day 23. Treasure Hunt

Day 24. So into You

Day 25. Dog on a Leash

Day 26. Bank on It

Day 27. Recharging Your
Batteries

Day 28. Driving on the
Shoulder

Day 29. Mirror Image

Day 30. I'm Feline Good

A Bone to Pick with You

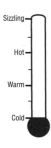

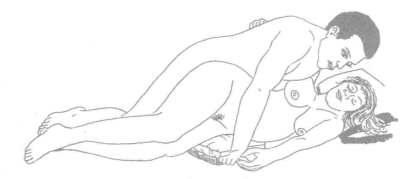

Or more accurately, a boner to pick you with! This sideways variation of the standard missionary position feels great!

Guys, you're sunny-side up on this one. Use a standard missionary pose with your arms in front of you and your legs straight behind you to achieve penetration.

Ladies, lie on your back with a pillow or two under your hips to elevate them. Your legs should be together and to one side of your partner. You'll need to twist your hips to the side or penetration will not be possible.

This position has a rather unique angle of penetration. Elevating the hips, even just a few inches, will change the tilt of the vagina and allow for deeper penetration. Having both of the woman's legs to the same side of the man's body means the man's penis is bumping up against the side of the vagina instead of the front or the back. Not only does this make the vagina feel a lot different, sideways positions are usually tighter too. Ladies, clench your vaginal muscles as your partner nears orgasm. The extra stimulation will send him over the top!

Bench Presses

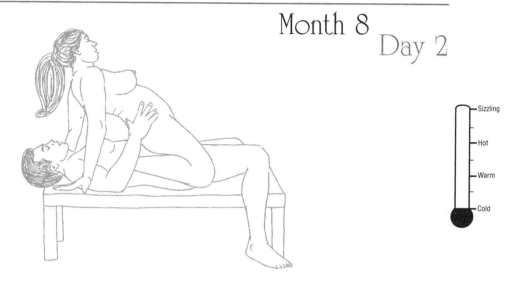

Sizzling

Hot

Warm

Cold

The bench is normally the spot for the B team and the subs. But not with this position. The prime-time players are on the bench tonight!

Guys, lie down on a bench or coffee table with your legs straddling the sides. For good thrusting, your feet need to reach the floor. Have your partner sit on top of you facing your feet. Her legs should be bent so that her feet are behind her. Once you've guided your penis inside, have her put her arms behind her and lean backward. Did you notice how much deeper it feels now?

Reach up and tickle your partner's neck. Run your fingers through her hair. Lightly tap your fingers along her spine from her neck all the way to her bottom. Stroke her sides from her hips to her armpits. Massage the skin on her arms from her shoulders down to her wrists or as far as you can comfortably reach.

Ladies, rock your hips backward and forward along your partner's shaft. You control the depth. Do a couple of shallow thrusts followed by a deep thrust. Continue alternating between shallow and deep until you can tell your partner is nearly climaxing. Then, let him stay deep inside of you until he orgasms.

Being benched has never been this much fun!

In Your Face

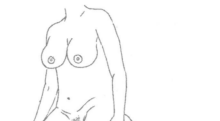

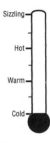

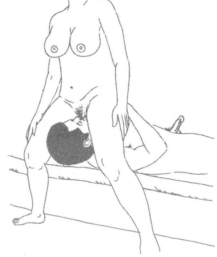

No matter how many people get in your face and ruin your day, when your partner gets in your face with this cunnilingus position, it'll make your night!

Guys, lie on your back with your head at the edge of the bed. Your partner should stand next to the bed facing away from your body. Have her straddle you so that her vulva is directly in your face. Use your hands to lower her hips into position.

Start by pointing your tongue and licking around the outside of the vagina. Using your tongue to poke the vaginal area produces a very pleasant sensation that is a little sharper than when a flat tongue is used. Insert just the tip of your tongue inside your partner's vagina. Rub it up against the very sensitive nerve endings that exist near the vaginal opening.

Use your tongue to separate her labia as you move your mouth up to the clitoral area. Flatten your tongue and rub it all over the clitoris and the surrounding skin and lips. Close your lips around the clitoris and rub your tongue back and forth. Feel her hips grinding into your face as she reaches her peak.

Shop Till You Pop

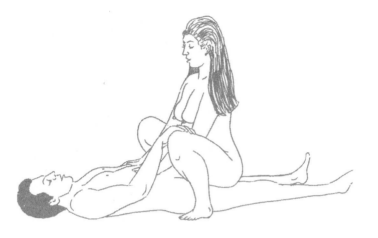

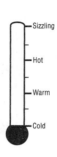

Sizzling

Hot

Warm

Cold

Attention all shoppers. This is a 24-hour one-stop shopping center where everybody can take care of their needs and desires.

Ladies, start out your shopping in the meat department. Have your partner lie on his back with his legs straight in front of him. His meat should be firm and fresh. Sit down on top facing him. Your legs should be bent with your feet flat on the bed next to his hips. Make sure you're warm and wet. Use your hand to help put his meat into your cart. Reach your hand between your partner's legs behind you and check out his ripe plums.

Guys, you get to visit the candy aisle. Use your hand to stimulate that sweet sticky spot between her legs. Rub your fingers back and forth until you feel her melt. Then, continue thrusting your hips until you have finished bagging your groceries.

Ladies, be careful getting up off your partner. We don't want a wet cleanup in aisle eight.

Complimentary Angles

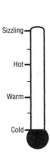

Sizzling —

Hot —

Warm —

Cold —

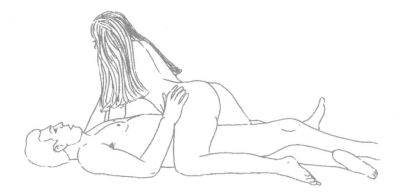

Complementary angles add up to ninety degrees. Complimentary angles add up to a lot of fun and pleasure!

For this position, the man is lying on his back with his legs straight in front of him. Ladies, you will be lying on top of your partner at a 45 degree angle to his shoulder. Your legs should be straight behind you with one of your legs entwined with one of your partner's legs. Rest your upper body weight on your arms in front of you. With your pubic bone bumped up against your partner's hips, you definitely want to initiate some grinding action.

Turn this into a complimentary angle. Make eye contact with each other and say something positive and sincere. "You're such a great lover" is okay. "I love to feel you deep inside of me when I orgasm" is much better. Everyone loves to be told that they're terrific. And the nice compliments we hear nicely complement the wonderful physical sensations we feel. It will enhance your lovemaking and increase the depth of your orgasm.

Touch of Class

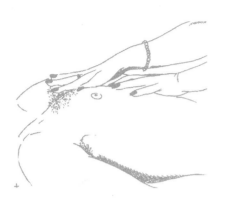

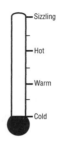

Sizzling

Hot

Warm

Cold

Ladies, this is an activity for you to manually stimulate your partner. It involves massaging your partner from his head to his genitals. It can be done in any position. I recommend having your partner lie on his back with you sitting on his hips.

Start by scratching his scalp. It's such a thick surface, but it's full of nerve endings. Friends I know claim that if they win the lottery they would hire someone to come to their house every day to give them a scalp massage while washing their hair. It just feels so good.

Move on and give him a facial massage. Rub your fingertips in circles from his forehead along his cheeks and to the bottom of his chin. Stroke your fingers back over the same areas. It'll give the impression of smoothing them out. Gently tickle your fingers up and down his neck. Use both hands to massage his chest and shoulders. Flatten your hands and use a full stroke up and down. With one finger, tease his nipples until they get hard.

Move back so that you are sitting on his thighs instead of his hips. Rub your hands down his stomach. Stroke your hands down each side of the V that is formed from his hipbones to his penis. Wrap your hands around his penis shaft.

Scoot yourself all the way forward so that you are sitting with his penis between your upper thighs. It works best if your legs are bent with your feet behind you. Squeeze your legs together while your hand is wrapped around the shaft. Rub the head against your clitoris. Your hand should use a full stroking motion from the base of the penis to the head and back down again. If your partner likes more pressure, tighten your grip around the shaft. Continue to stroke him until he's climaxed.

Winner's Circle

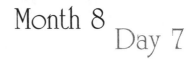

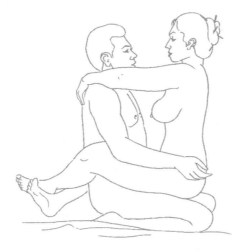

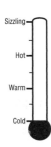

Sizzling

Hot

Warm

Cold

With her legs wrapped around your waist, you'll feel like you are in the winner's circle with this position.

Guys, kneel down with your legs completely bent so that you're practically sitting on the back of your calves. Have your partner sit on your lap facing you. In order for you to penetrate, she'll need to sit very close to you. Have her wrap her legs around your waist.

Focus on the intimacy of the position. Brush your lips up against her neck and ear. It'll be pleasantly ticklish. Very chastely, kiss her on the lips. It's a definite tease because you know she wants more. Kiss her with your lips opened. Wait for her tongue to come looking for yours. Enjoy some passionate kisses with your lover.

Put your hands on her breasts while you're kissing her. Let the actions of your hands mirror the intensity of the kisses. Start by just brushing your hands up against her breasts. Then use your fingers to toy with her nipples. Finally, rub the nipples with the palms of your hands while your fingers are massaging the rest of the breasts.

Help your partner reach her peak, and a return trip to the winner's circle is guaranteed.

Cream of the Crop

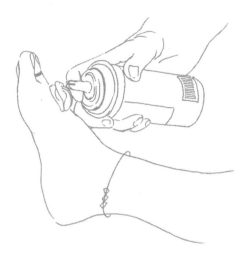

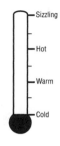

Sizzling

Hot

Warm

Cold

Whipped cream, that is. So, get out the can of whipped fun for this cunnilingus activity!

Start with the feet. Spray the whipped cream along the bottom of your partner's foot, particularly around the arch. The cold, wet, smooth texture has a unique feeling. Use your tongue to lick it off. The ticklish feeling of your rough tongue and the smooth cream is highly arousing!

Have your partner roll onto her stomach. For most women, the back of the leg is much more sensitive than the front, so apply the whipped cream to the back of her leg from her ankle to her buttocks. Use a little extra on the back of the knee and the top of the thigh. These seem to be favorite erogenous spots for many women. Use your tongue and lips to explore your partner's legs. Find out your partner's most sensitive spots and remember them for the future.

Before moving onto your partner's genitals, have her roll onto her back and spread her legs apart. Spray whipped cream on your partner's labia from her clitoris down to her vagina. She will love the way the cold whipped cream feels on her hot vulva! Rub your tongue back and forth on her skin as you lick it clean. Apply some additional whipped cream on the clitoral area. Close your mouth around the area and suck on it. Rub your tongue back and forth over her sweet clitoris.

When she's finished with her orgasms, she'll know for certain that you are the cream of the crop!

One-Night Stand

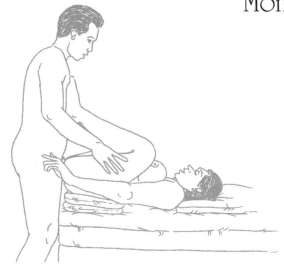

Sizzling
Hot
Warm
Cold

This is a stand-alone position for the man that will definitely stand the test of time. So let's not stand on ceremony. Let's get started.

Ladies, lie on your back with your legs over the edge of the bed. In order for your partner to stand a chance of penetrating, bend your knees to your chest and rest your feet against your partner's chest. It stands to reason that your chances of experiencing an orgasm will increase if you use your hand to stimulate your clitoris.

Guys, stand up next to the bed. Lean against your partner's feet, insert the head of your penis into her vagina, and thrust your hips forward. The depth of this position will make your hair stand on end. There is no need to stand still. Continue thrusting your hips until neither of you can stand it any longer!

Use the position regularly and make it a long-standing tradition.

Down and Dirty

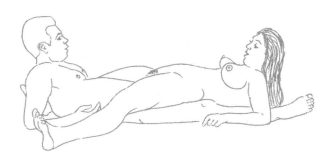

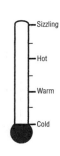

Before starting this position, get each other hot and wet by reading some erotic material to each other. If you can write your own, great! You definitely get some bonus points. Otherwise, look in magazines, books, or on the Internet and find something you think is steamy. Read your selections out loud to each other. You might feel a bit uncomfortable when you start, but once you get into it, you'll find it very arousing.

And so will your partner!

For this position, both of you will be reclining on your back with your arms bent behind you and your weight on your elbows. Ladies, start out by sitting on top of your partner with your legs spread open wide. Once his penis is enjoying your wonderful wetness, lean backward. If you can support your weight on one arm, use the other hand to massage your breasts. Gently pull on the nipple. This is arousing

for you and a great visual treat for your partner.

Guys, use one of your hands to manually stimulate your partner. Let her set the rhythm and pace by letting her rock her hips up against your hand. For many women, this little bit of control significantly improves their chances of experiencing an orgasm. Have her continue to thrust her hips until you've reached your peak too.

The Corkscrew

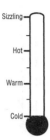

Sizzling

Hot

Warm

Cold

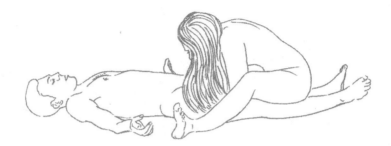

Get out the corkscrew for this fellatio position! Come on guys, relax! She's just using it to open a bottle of wine to help set the mood. What were you thinking?

Ladies, have your partner lie on his back with his legs straight in front of him. Sit down on his thighs. This will give you a great angle, and is also a pleasant means of preventing your partner from squirming. Men love to be physically pinned down by their partner. (It's pinning them

down mentally and emotionally that some of them can't handle!)

Try to distract your partner's attention by rubbing your hands on his stomach and hips. When he's not looking, lean forward and put your mouth around the head and shaft of his penis. The unexpected pleasure of your warm and wet mouth will be like a jolt of electricity running through him. They love it!

Lift and lower your

head up and down the shaft of your partner's penis. Use a twisting motion with your head each time you raise and lower it. The corkscrew motion alters which part of your mouth and tongue are on each part of his penis. This minor motion significantly increases the intensity, so don't be surprised if his orgasm comes a little quicker than usual!

Every Dog Has His Day

Month 8
Day 12

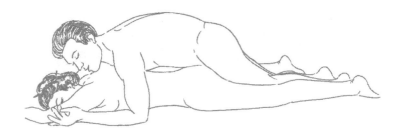

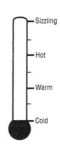

And today is yours!

This is a slight variation of the standard doggy-style position. Both of you start on your hands and knees with the woman in front so the man can enter her from behind. Penetration is usually easier if the woman's legs are on the outside of the man's legs. After penetration has occurred, both of you should lean forward together. Couples that don't synchronize this will lose penetration. The woman should lean all the way forward so that her arms and chest are flat against the bed. Her hips and bottom should still be arched up. The man should lean forward far enough to rest his upper body weight on his elbows. He does not lie flat against his partner for this position.

Ladies, even with your arms flat, you can still reach back and manually stimulate your clitoris. Most women experience significant vaginal stimulation with rear-entry positions. These sensations are heightened when you masturbate simultaneously. Try to match the tempo of your partner's thrusts so you can reach your peaks at the same time.

Dancing on Tables

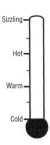

Sizzling

Hot

Warm

Cold

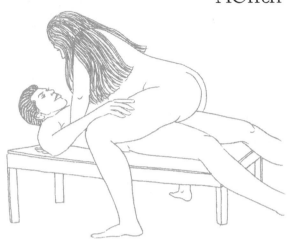

Ladies, now it's your turn to do a striptease dance on the coffee table for your partner. For the best view, have him sit on the floor. Slowly and seductively remove each item of clothing and drop it on your partner's lap. When you've removed your panties, keep your legs spread open while you dance around. His seat from the floor lets him see everything! He'll be very aroused watching you.

Now it's time to use the coffee table for some horizontal dancing. Have your partner lie down on his back with his legs opened wide on the table. Climb on top of your partner, facing him, with your feet straddling the table. Start by rubbing your vulva against one of his thighs. The soft feel of your hot and silky skin drives him crazy, and will feel great to you too!

Lift up your hips so that your partner's penis just barely touches the entrance to your vagina. Tease him by letting just the tip of his penis touch you while you wiggle your hips and dance around. Finally, let him inside by lowering yourself down his shaft.

Lean all the way forward. Let your tongues dance together as you give your partner a kiss. Let your breasts dance against his chest. Rock your hips until your partner is too exhausted to dance any longer.

Face the Music

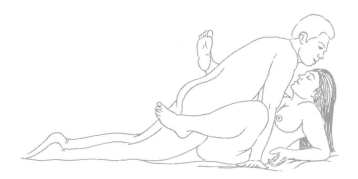

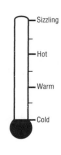

Strike up the band! We're ready to make some music! Only duets allowed with this position. You'll have to find some other time to play your instrument solo.

Guys, since you have the baton, you can be the conductor. Have your partner lie on her back with her arms bent behind her and her weight on her elbows. Encourage her to shimmy her shoulders and shake her maracas on the way down. You'll be plucking her strings from the standard missionary pose.

Ladies, once his drumstick starts beating a rhythm inside of you, bend one leg so that your foot is sideways by his hips. Wrap your other leg around his waist. Be sure your hips are matching the same tempo as his thrusts. Playing a sharp instead of a flat can ruin the tune!

The key to making great music is to read the notes. Watch for signals that indicate whether your partner is close to reaching his peak. When he is, increase the tempo and bring the concert to a resounding finish.

Best Seat in the House

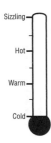

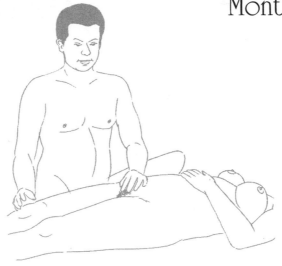

Guys, this is a position where you manually stimulate your partner. So have her lie down on her back and get comfortable. Then sit down next to her.

Spread her legs apart, but don't stimulate her genitals yet. Use your fingernails and lightly scratch the skin on her thighs. This is meant to be stimulating; it's not meant to hurt or leave a mark. It's a light touch with fingernails instead of fingertips. Tap your fingers against the inside of her thighs. Stroke the skin above and around her pubic hair.

Run your fingers through her pubic hair, gently pulling some of them. Gradually work your way to her vulva. Rub a finger around the outside of your partner's vagina, spreading around the lubrication. Move your finger to her clitoral area and rub the hood back and forth over her clitoris.

Leaving your hand where it is, lean your upper body sideways so that your mouth can reach her breasts. Many women love to have their breasts stimulated while their clitoris is being rubbed. Put your mouth around the entire nipple. Have your tongue rub the nipple back and forth at the same speed that your fingers are rubbing her clitoris. Enjoy the view from your seat as she arches her back and climaxes.

Mixed Nuts

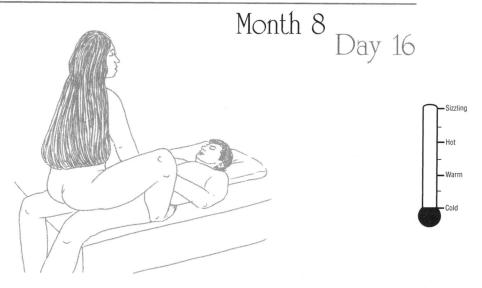

Sizzling

Hot

Warm

Cold

Whether you like hazelnuts, walnuts, cashews, or almonds, you'll love what we do to nuts in this position!

Guys, lie on your back with your legs hanging over the edge of the bed.

Ladies, spread your partner's legs apart and stand between them. Lean over and give his nuts a lick. Rub your tongue back and forth between them. Open your

mouth and fully surround one of his nuts with your lips. Now lick the nut from inside of your mouth!

Sit down on top of your partner facing him. Let his penis slide into you as you lower yourself onto him. Bend your legs so that your feet will be sideways by your partner's hips. Reach behind you and wrap your hand around his testicles. Jostle them, roll them,

squeeze them. But be gentle. They can be very sensitive. We're not trying to make peanut butter!

Let your partner do most of the thrusting for this position. As you feel him starting to reach his peak, wrap two fingers around the base of his penis. The additional stimulation is guaranteed to drive him nuts!

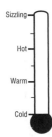

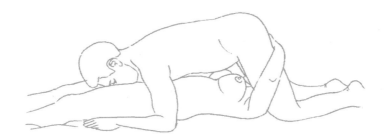

And, I don't mean at a restaurant!

No need to rush to the main entrée. Start with some slow sweet kisses. We use our lips to explore so many body parts that we sometimes forget the simple pleasures of basic lip-to-lip kissing.

For the next course, the woman should lie on her back with her legs spread apart. The man kneels by the woman's head and leans forward to kiss and nibble her breasts. While he is enjoying this delightfully tasty treat, the woman should kiss, lick, suck, and tickle his torso.

When you're finally hungry enough for the main course, the man should fully straddle his partner, allowing her to wrap her lips around his penis while he manipulates his tongue all around her vulva. Use your lips, tongue, and teeth to slowly build up your partner's arousal. Take turns finishing off the meal with a climactic dessert.

If your stomach is still growling for food, go eat out at a restaurant. When you get home, you can eat out again.

Knock on Woody

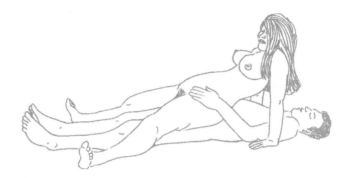

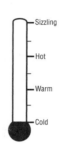

You're not superstitious, but somehow you just can't resist the urge to knock on wood when you need to ward off some bad luck. I think this custom would be greatly improved if instead of knocking our hand against wood, we knocked our hand or our hips against a woody. That would help us forget about any potential bad luck!

The man lies on his back with his legs straight in front of him. Ladies, rub your hand up and down your partner's woody to check for splinters. Use your tongue to sand down any rough spots.

Wrap your hand around your partner's trunk and guide it inside of your vagina as you sit down on your partner facing his feet.

Your legs should be spread open wide. Put your arms behind you and lean backward. This gives the tree lots more room to grow! Rest your weight on one arm so that you can use one hand to manually stimulate your clitoris. Knock your hips against his woody until both of you orgasm.

Sitting Pretty

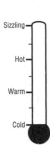

Sizzling

Hot

Warm

Cold

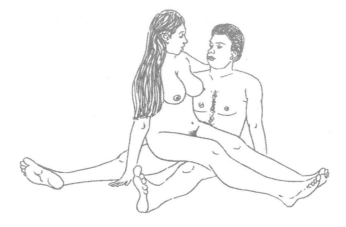

Not only does your partner look pretty, she's also sitting pretty with this position that puts her in your lap. So, fellas, sit on the bed with your legs spread apart in front of you. Have your partner sit down sideways in your lap. As she lowers her hips, use your hand to guide your penis into her vagina. Depending on her size, she might need for you to put a pillow under her bottom to help hold her up once penetration has been achieved.

Enjoy the closeness of this position. Rub the palm of your hand against your partner's nipples while you kiss her on the neck. Kiss the base of her neck and then drag your tongue down to her breasts. Very lightly rub your lips against her breasts. This can be more arousing than when her breasts are fully massaged. Put your arms around your partner and hold her tight while you reach your peak.

Growing Season

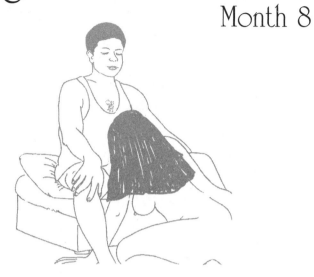

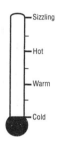

Everyone knows that you need lots of water to make things grow. Ladies, this fellatio activity starts before your partner is erect, so you might need to wait until a time when he's not expecting it.

For a few of you, the challenge will be finding a time when your partner isn't already thinking about sex. For the rest of us, this requirement is not too difficult. Your best chances for success are probably when he's watching TV. However, if you have a devilish streak in you, try this while he's talking on the phone. It's particularly effective if he's talking to his parents or someone from work!

No need for foreplay with this activity. In fact, foreplay will simply make him hard and end your growing season prematurely. Walk up to your partner, unzip his pants, pull out his penis, and put the entire thing into your mouth. This is an incredible rush for guys! The combination of being taken by surprise plus the sensations from your hot, wet mouth will feel like an electric current running through his body. Rub your tongue all around the head and the shaft. As he becomes more aroused, let the head and shaft of his penis slide into and out of your mouth. Increase the stimulation by putting your hand around the shaft and moving it up and down simultaneously with your mouth. He'll be reaching his orgasm in no time!

Full-Court Press

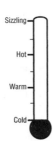

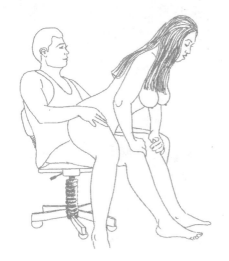

You have a courtside seat for this basketball game, guys, so make yourself comfortable in a chair or on the couch. Your partner will be facing away from you with her legs spread open and to the outside of your legs. Pull your partner down onto your lap and dunk one into her net. What a shot! Double-team your partner by moving both hands to the front to massage her breasts.

Ladies, lean your upper body forward as far as it will go. You'll receive a personal foul and might get ejected from the game if you do this too quickly and accidentally hurt your partner. Reach down with your hand and dribble the ball between his legs. If you're really good, do some double dribbling by massaging both balls in one hand at the same time. Continue running plays until his shot clock has expired.

Tongue in Cheek

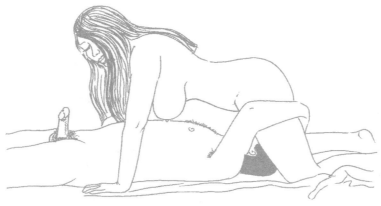

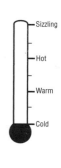

Sizzling

Hot

Warm

Cold

And in many other places too!

This is a great cunnilingus position. The man lies on his back. His partner straddles him so that her head is facing his feet.

Guys, grasp your partner's hips and pull her warm and wonderful vulva to your face. Put your tongue between her cheeks and lick the tender skin around the entrance of the vagina. Insert your tongue into her vagina. Have your partner lift and lower her hips while you move your tongue all around inside of her with each thrust.

Pull your partner's hips backward so that your tongue can reach her clitoris. Flatten your tongue and make the entire area nice and wet. Seal your lips around her clitoris and hum a happy tune. Women love this! It turns your mouth into a miniature vibrator! Rub your tongue back and forth until she has as many orgasms as she can handle!

Treasure Hunt

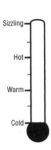

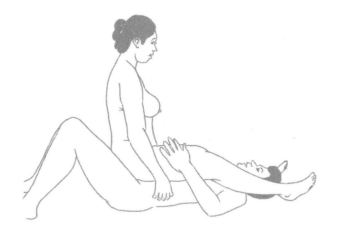

Ladies, set the scenario so your partner can hunt for and find your valuable treasures. Hang a pair of panties on the doorknob for when he gets home. Attach a sexy and seductive note letting him know where to find the next hint. Create a trail of lingerie, sex toys, erotic pictures, and any other items that remind your partner of sex and eventually lead him to your

bedroom. Be there waiting for him. He has found his treasure!

Have your partner lie on his back with his legs bent at the knees. Lean over and polish his jewels with your tongue. Sit on top of him, inserting his valuable treasure into your treasure box. Put your legs straight in front of you on his shoulders. This will keep your treasure box nice and

tight and prevent his jewels from falling out. Use your hands to massage your treasure chest. Rub your nipples between your fingers, letting your partner watch and enjoy. As your partner's arousal increases and he starts approaching his peak, put your hand behind you and squeeze the base of his penis with two of your fingers. His hunt for the treasure will soon be over!

So into You

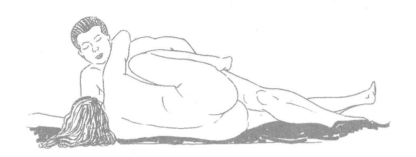

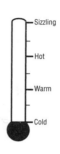

- Sizzling
- Hot
- Warm
- Cold

This is a very intimate side-by-side position that is great for a night of tenderness, love, and romance.

Most couples find it difficult to achieve penetration if they start out lying next to each other. Instead, establish penetration by having the woman sit on top of the man facing toward him.

Then, have her lean forward and extend her legs backward so that she is lying on him. At that point, the man should hold his partner very tight and roll them both onto their sides. Move the legs a bit to make them more comfortable. The woman should have one leg under her partner's leg. To increase the depth of penetration, her other leg

should be bent and pressed up to her chest. Voilà! You are now comfortably in a side-by-side position!

Enjoy the face-to-face closeness this position offers. Kiss and cuddle. Stroke your partner's hair, face, and neck. Whisper to each other about how totally and completely in love you are. Hold your partner tight as you climax.

Dog on a Leash

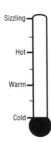

Sizzling

Hot

Warm

Cold

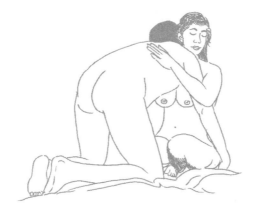

Woof! Woof! Your partner will be barking in pleasure while you manually stimulate him in this position.

Ladies, sit cross-legged on the bed or floor. Have your partner on his hands and knees, doggy-style, in front of you. Reach underneath him and rub your hands on his chest. Put your arms around him and give him a squeeze before you run your hands down his back. Bring your hands around to the front and work your way to his genitals.

Guys, you've got your head right next to your partner's shoulder. Nibble her ears and kiss her neck. Whisper in her ear how much you love what she's doing.

Ladies, the stroking technique for this position works best with lubrication. The hands need to slide easily along the penis. Use some oil, lotion, or saliva to get things wet. Wrap your right hand around the shaft of your partner's penis and stroke it. Start at the

bottom and let your hand go all the way off the top. Now, wrap your left hand around the shaft and do the same thing. Continue alternating between right and left, starting each stroke at the bottom and letting the hand go completely off the top. When his tongue starts hanging out and you hear him panting, you'll know he's close to reaching his peak. Rub one hand up and down the shaft and head until he orgasms.

Bank on It

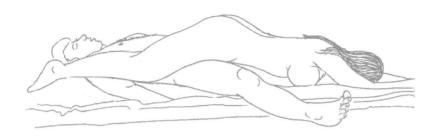

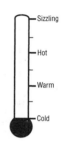

Sizzling

Hot

Warm

Cold

Don't use the ATM for this transaction. You need a live teller! This position has a high interest rate and yields great returns.

Guys, lie on your back with your legs spread open. Make sure you have a stiff roll of quarters to work with. A couple of crumpled-up dollar bills won't do the trick.

Ladies, position your hips over the head of your partner's penis. You need to be facing his feet. Use your hand to guide his valuables into your safety deposit box. Once securely locked into place, extend your legs straight behind you and lean forward so that your arms and chest are resting on the bed.

Guys, this position is not very deep, so thrust carefully. Remember, you must maintain a minimum balance and will incur a penalty for an early withdrawal. Continue thrusting your hips until you have made a deposit into your partner's account.

Recharging Your Batteries

Month 8
Day 27

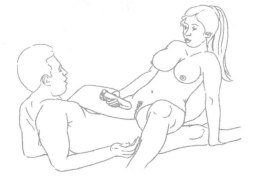

Sizzling

Hot

Warm

Cold

In this activity the woman uses a vibrator on herself during intercourse. But, before you choose a position, you need to know where the vibrator is going to be used.

If the woman uses the vibrator to stimulate her clitoris, then you have a wide variety of positions from which to choose. In man-on-top positions and those where the woman lies on the man, the clitoris is not accessible. On the other hand, positions where the woman is sitting on top of the man work great with the vibrator — especially when the woman has her legs spread wide open. Doggy-style positions are also very useful. These are all very stimulating for most women, so the vibrator turns a good position into a great one.

A woman can also use the vibrator anally. It's a little more challenging to find intercourse positions that allow the woman to insert the vibrator in her anus. Anal penetration is also more difficult to achieve than stimulating the clitoris. But the overwhelming intensity of the sensations makes the effort worthwhile. Almost all positions that have either the man or woman lying at an angle to their partner will work as well.

If you're having difficulty finding a position that will work, use one of the suggestions below.

When the woman uses the vibrator during sex, it does more than just increase the intensity of the intercourse for her. It also enhances the sexual experience for her partner. Whether she uses the vibrator on her clitoris or her anus, the man will feel the vibrations on his penis while it's inside her vagina. His sensations are not as strong as the woman's, but they are certainly very, very pleasant!

Suggested positions: Month 1/Day 18 — Sidesaddle; Month 5/Day 7 — The Catbird Seat; Month 7/Day 13 — War and Peace; Month 8/Day 12 — Every Dog Has His Day; Month 11/Day 21 — Horsing Around; Month 12/Day 6 — Happy Hour.

Driving on the Shoulder

Month 8
Day 28

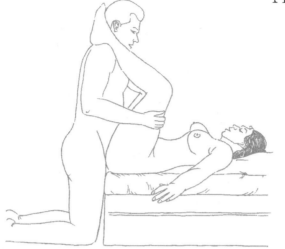

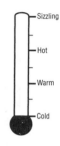

- Sizzling
- Hot
- Warm
- Cold

Guys, don't give your partner the cold shoulder! She needs somewhere to rest her warm legs, and your broad shoulders are just the place!

Have your partner lie on her back with her legs over the edge of the bed. In order for you to be able to penetrate, she needs to have her bottom all the way to the edge. You will be kneeling on the floor with your thighs pressed up against the side of the bed. Help your partner lift her legs up onto your shoulders, then insert your penis into her vagina, and thrust your hips forward. Having her legs up makes this position particularly deep. So start out using long, deep, slow thrusts. As your arousal increases, your thrusts will become quicker and shallower.

Reach in front of you and massage your partner's breasts. Encourage your partner to show you what she likes. Have her use one of her hands on one breast while you use one of your hands on her other breast. Take notice of how she uses her fingers, which parts of the breast she likes to have stimulated the most, and how much pressure to use. Each woman's needs are unique. She'll be most appreciative when you're able to meet hers.

Mirror Image

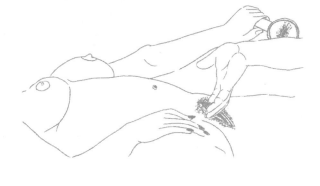

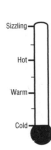

Sizzling

Hot

Warm

Cold

Guys, you know how much you love to watch your partner stimulating you by hand. Part of the attraction is watching the palm of her hand rub against the head of your penis, or her fingers wrapped around your shaft. With this activity, your partner can watch while you manually stimulate her. A woman cannot see a finger going into her vagina or rubbing on her clitoris. The entire visual dimension of sex is completely lost. So, you need to have a mirror ready for her.

Choose a position where observation will be possible.

If she lies on her back with her legs spread open, she can hold a mirror in her hand and move it around to see her entire vulva. A second option is to put a wall mirror on the floor. Have your partner assume the hands and knees doggy-style position over the mirror. You kneel behind her with your arms wrapped around her. She can watch everything by looking down into the mirror below her. If you don't have a mirror to put on the floor, find a wall mirror she can sit in front of. A bathroom mirror works if the counter is wide enough

for her to sit comfortably. Have your partner sit in front of the mirror with her legs bent and spread open. The closer she sits to the mirror, the more she'll see. You stand or sit behind her and reach your hand around or under her leg.

Once you have your partner and the mirror set up, let her see how you stimulate her. Rub around and inside her vagina. Spread apart her labia and rub the lips between your thumb and finger. Rub your fingers against her clitoris. The visual stimulation will intensify her orgasm.

I'm Feline Good

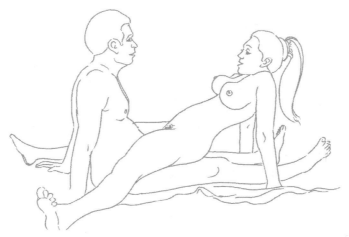

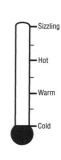

Sizzling

Hot

Warm

Cold

Watch out, guys. Cats are carnivores, and you know what that means. They love to eat your meat! So it's time to give your partner's pussycat a little treat.

Guys, sit down on the bed with your legs straight in front of you. Have your partner sit on your lap facing you with her legs spread wide behind you. Hold the shaft of your penis and guide it inside your partner as she lowers herself into your lap. Once you've established penetration, have your partner put her arms behind her and lean backward against them.

Use your hand to rub your partner's pubic hair. Scratch your fingers on the skin underneath it. Gently tug and pull it. Turn your hand so that your palm is on your partner's pubic hair and your fingers are on her clitoris. While pushing down with your palm, rub her clitoris back and forth with your fingers. Let her thrusting hips set the pace. Continue stimulating her until she's used up her nine lives!

Interested in trying new things to see if they're right for you and your partner? Go right ahead. Curiosity didn't really kill the cat!

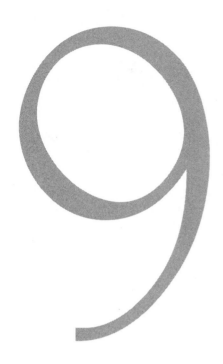

MONTH 9

Day 1. Come Unglued

Day 2. Hard Candy

Day 3. Standing at Attention

Day 4. Diamond in the

Rough

Day 5. Reading Braille

Day 6. Certified Pubic

Accountant

Day 7. The Boss

Day 8. Stick It to You

Day 9. Lap of Luxury

Day 10. Sleight of Hand

Day 11. Forecasting Fun

Day 12. Squeaky Clean

Day 13. Heart to Heart

Day 14. Great Sexpectations

Day 15. Self-Indulgence

Day 16. Talk the Talk

Day 17. Falling for You

Day 18. Fire Down Below

Day 19. Lateral Thinking

Day 20. Puck You!

Day 21. Tongue Twisters

Day 22. Sideshow

Day 23. Good Vibrations

Day 24. The Texas Two-Step

Day 25. On Bended Knees

Day 26. Rub You the

Right Way

Day 27. The Dirty Deed

Day 28. Head Coach

Day 29. Body Chemistry

Day 30. Split the Difference

Come Unglued

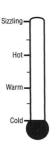

Sizzling
Hot
Warm
Cold

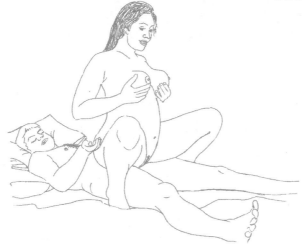

Let me come straight to the point. This position will definitely have you coming back for more!

The man lies on his back with his legs spread apart. Ladies, don't be afraid to come on too strong. In fact, your partner will be happy if you let things come to blows. Lower your mouth over his penis and feel it come to life. Straddle your partner facing his feet. Your legs should be bent so that your feet are flat on the floor next to his hips. Lift your hips and come down so that your partner's penis can slide into your vagina. Clench your vaginal muscles. You don't want his penis to accidentally come out.

Put your hand between your legs. A little masturbation will certainly come in handy right about now. Don't let anything come between you and your partner. Once everything has come up roses for both of you, you can come to a halt.

We'll definitely come again soon!

Hard Candy

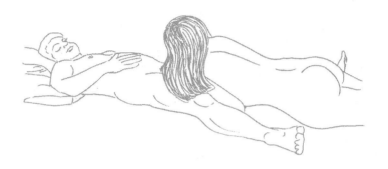

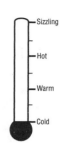

Sizzling

Hot

Warm

Cold

Ladies, this is a fellatio position that will have your mouth watering! Have your partner lie on his back with his stick of candy straight in the air. Spread his legs apart and lie on your tummy between them. I think you know what to do with hard candy. You suck it!

Put your mouth around the head of your partner's penis and get it wet. Stick your tongue out of your mouth and lick the head of his penis like a lollipop. Watching your tongue against his penis is eye candy for your partner. Very arousing! Wrap your hand around the shaft and lower your mouth back over the entire penis head. Let your hand move up and down the shaft while your tongue continues to lick around the head. And remember, it's bad for your teeth to chew on hard candy. So continue sucking until the candy dissolves.

Standing at Attention

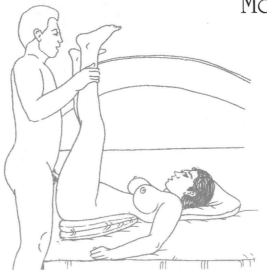

Sizzling

Hot

Warm

Cold

Guys, you will be standing at attention next to the bed for this position. Make sure your troops are standing at attention too before you get started.

Stand in front of your partner, who is lying on her back with her legs over the edge of the bed. If you're very tall, you'll need to put a pillow or two under your partner's hips so you can penetrate. Lift up her legs and hold them together straight in front of you. Move your hips so that the tip of your penis is lined up with the entrance of your partner's vagina. Slowly thrust your hips forward and let your entire penis slide inside of her.

Stroke your partner's calves and knees with your hands. Lean forward and rub your nose against the bottom of her foot. Suck on your partner's toes. Feet and ankles can be highly erogenous. Explore them with your hands, lips, and tongue. Make sure your partner gives you feedback to help you find the best spots and techniques to make her happy.

This is a very deep and tight position. Continue thrusting your hips until you've reached your peak.

Diamond in the Rough

Month 9
Day 4

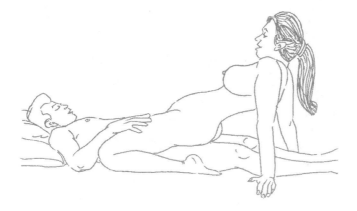

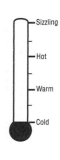

Diamonds, the hardest known mineral, are formed under intense pressure and heat. So ladies, use your heat to determine if your partner's got a diamond between his legs or just a cubic zirconia.

Start with a visual examination. Get it wet with your tongue so it can shine brilliantly in the light. Rub your hand along the shaft to make sure it's hard and solid. Sit on your partner, facing him, with your legs bent so that your feet are behind you. Use your hand to guide his diamond into your jewelry box. Put your arms behind you and lean backward. Feel how the penetration just got a lot tighter.

Lean back on just one arm and use the other hand to masturbate. Spread your knees apart as wide as they will go. Not only does this give you more room to maneuver your hand, it also makes the penetration for your partner much deeper. Rub your fingers back and forth and all around your clitoris. It's okay if you orgasm before your partner. Just continue thrusting your hips until his diamond has finished sparkling.

No wonder diamonds are a girl's best friend.

Reading Braille

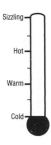

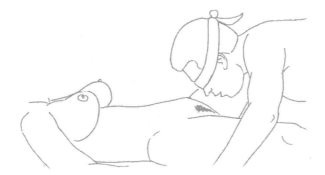

Guys, this is a cunnilingus activity where you, not your partner, are blindfolded. You'll have to rely on your fingers and your tongue to find the right spots that will bring her to orgasm. So put on your blindfold and let's get started.

Begin the activity with a little hide-and-seek foreplay. She hides. You seek. Have your partner give you little hints as to where she is. After all, it's in her best interests for you to find her. Once you've found her, undress her. For guys who

struggle to undress their partner when they can see, this could prove to be a challenge while they're blindfolded. Enjoy it! Have fun! There is nothing wrong with a good laugh. Kiss and nibble each part of her body as you undress it.

Position your partner and yourself so you can find her vulva with your hands and mouth. Pretend you can't find the right spot. Start at her feet and slowly caress and kiss your way up her legs until you get to the top. From there, let your tongue

take over. Point your tongue and tickle the tops of her thighs. Rub the side of your tongue up between the labia. Flatten your tongue and rub it back and forth against the clitoris. Listen to the sounds she makes as her arousal increases. Let your hands feel her body responding to your tongue. When you've found a spot that gets a great response, continue to stimulate it with your tongue until she reaches her peak.

Certified Pubic Accountant

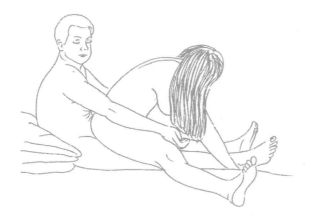

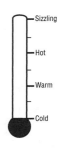

Sizzling

Hot

Warm

Cold

You don't have to be a bean counter to love this position! It's an acquisition and merger that will reap big profits.

Guys, sit down with your legs straight in front of you. Lower your partner down onto your lap, facing away from you. Her legs should be spread open wide. Use your hand to guide your capital into her accounts receivable. To be in positional compliance, your partner should lean all the way forward.

Put your hands on your partner's wonderful ass-et. Massage her breasts with one hand while you massage her clitoris with the other. Continue thrusting until both of you have cashed in on your financial gains.

Most companies only generate financial statements every month or quarter. As a diligent CPA, you should be checking your accounts every day!

The Boss

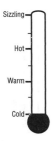

Sizzling —
Hot —
Warm —
Cold —

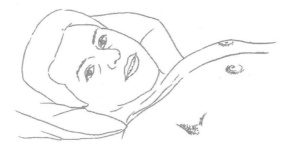

Ladies, let your partner be the boss. With this intercourse activity the man chooses where and when the sex will occur. He also gets to choose the foreplay and the position. Of course, all of this requires a degree of reasonability to be applied. Sometimes men get to make a few choices and get totally carried away. On the front lawn at noon does not qualify as acceptable. And, no, this is not his big chance to invite your best friend to join you.

This activity is not about power. The purpose of this activity is to find out what really makes your partner tick. Does he prefer sex before work? Does he like oral sex as foreplay? Does he prefer positions where he can stimulate your clitoris or positions where he can watch you masturbate? Does he like the penetration to be tight, deep, or both? This is a chance to explore your partner's preferences. Learning more about each other will ultimately improve and enhance your sexual relationship together.

Stick It to You

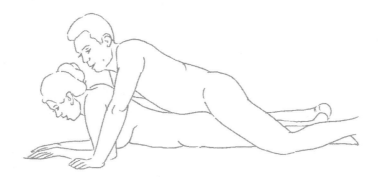

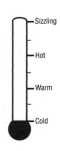

This is a rear-entry position that lets you stick it to your partner.

The easiest way to get penetration with this position is to start out in the standard hands-and-knees doggy-style position. Use your hand to guide your penis to her vagina.

Once you've successfully achieved penetration, both of you should extend your legs behind you. Make sure this is a coordinated effort. If not, you'll almost certainly be starting over. Have your partner lower her upper body so that her arms are bent and her weight is on her elbows. You should keep your arms straight and have your weight on your wrists.

To make the position even tighter than usual, move your legs so that they are outside your partner's legs. This will increase the intensity of the sensations both of you will feel, and increase your partner's chance of having an orgasm.

Lap of Luxury

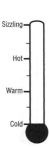

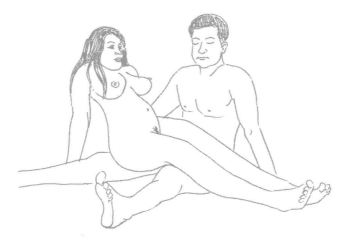

It doesn't matter how much money you have. You can sit in the lap of luxury when you use this position!

Ladies, have your partner sit on the bed or floor with his legs spread open. Start by using your mouth to make sure your partner is wet. You want him to slide right in. Sit down sideways on your partner's lap. Use your hand to help guide his penis into your hot, wet vagina. Squeeze your legs together in front of you. It makes the tight sideways penetration even tighter. Put your arms behind you and lean backward.

Guys, this is a great chance to show your partner how valuable she is to you. Start by caressing and stroking her breasts. Rub her nipples with your index fingers until they get taut. Then gently pull the nipple and rub it between your finger and thumb. Lightly drag your fingertips down your partner's torso from her breasts to her pubic hair. Rest your palm on your partner's pubic hair, while your fingers are on her clitoris. Push down with the palm of your hand while your fingers stimulate her clitoris. Increase the intensity of your thrusting as you feel your partner getting more and more aroused. Feel her back arch as she orgasms against your fingers.

Sleight of Hand

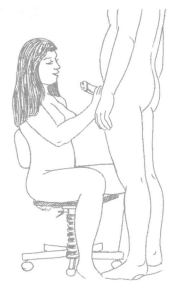

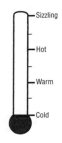

Sizzling

Hot

Warm

Cold

Your hand doesn't need to be faster than his eyes for your partner to feel the magic of this manual stimulation position!

Ladies, sit comfortably in a chair. Have your partner stand in front of you. This gives you a unique angle for stimulating him. Bend your head forward and drag your hair across your partner's penis. The soft, silky touch is extremely arousing. Reach down and wrap your hands around his testicles while continuing to stroke him with your hair.

Using just the tips of your fingers, stimulate the head of your partner's penis. Start with your fingers around the edge of the head and gently pull them to the center. Keep your thumb on the very sensitive slit on the underside of the head.

Wrap your hand around the shaft of your partner's penis. Pull your hand up the shaft and head toward you. Gently twist your hand from side to side as you move from the base to the head. This will cause very pleasant variations in the sensations your partner experiences. Be careful not to pull your partner's skin while you do this. Friction burns on the penis are not erotic! Use one hand to hold his testicles while your other hand continues stroking. Increase the pace and pressure until your partner reaches his peak.

Forecasting Fun

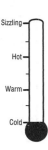

Sizzling
Hot
Warm
Cold

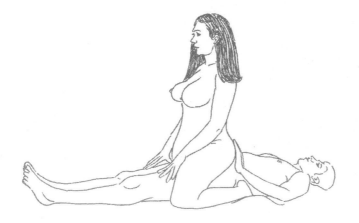

The weatherman is checking his satellite photos. He says to be prepared for some global warming!

Guys, lie on your back with your legs straight in front of you. Feel the warm front that moves into the area when your partner straddles you facing your feet. As she lifts her hips, place your hand underneath her and use your finger to make sure she's reached her dew point. If she has, she'll feel hot and humid! You don't need a weather map to guide your penis inside her vagina.

Ladies, your legs should be bent so that your feet are behind you. Create some turbulence in the atmosphere by thrusting your hips forward, backward, and around in a circle. Rub your hand against your clitoris. Let the humidity index continue to rise until both of you have reached your high temperatures for the day.

The forecast for this position is always very hot! Don't worry about contributing to the greenhouse effect. Feel free to crank up the heat as often as you want!

Squeaky Clean

Month 9
Day 12

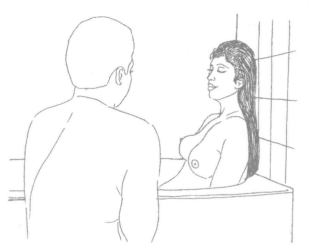

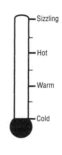

Okay, guys. Run warm water into the bathtub. Add some bubble bath. Light a candle. Pour your partner a glass of wine. Undress her and help her into the tub. This is your chance to give your partner a relaxing bubble bath that includes some manual stimulation.

Use a washcloth and cover your partner's shoulders and arms with warm soapy water. Put soap on your hands and massage her breasts. Notice how the skin and nipples get soft when they're wet. Lovingly rub soap all over your partner's body. Enjoy the smooth silkiness of her wet skin. Move your hand between your partner's legs. Use your finger to rub the area around her vagina. Let your slippery wet finger slide into and out of her slippery wet vagina. Move your fingers up to her labia. They will feel a bit swollen from being in the water. Let your fingers rub around the clitoral area. As your partner's arousal increases, lean over and put your mouth around her nipple while continuing to rub her clitoris at the same time. Continue stimulating her until she reaches her peak.

Once the bath is over, wrap your partner in a towel and help her dry off. It's a sweet touch that will score some bonus points for you!

Heart to Heart

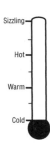

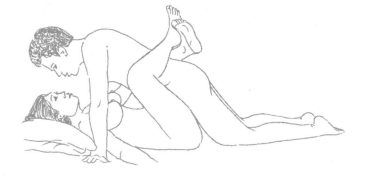

Although it's physically impossible for two people to actually lie heart to heart, this very intimate position gets you pretty close.

This is a common variation of the standard missionary position. Instead of having her legs straight in front of her on the bed, the woman wraps her legs around her partner's waist.

Not only does this allow for deeper penetration, it also helps generate a feeling of comfort, closeness, and security.

Enjoy the intimacy of being face-to-face with your partner. Feel your two hearts beat as one. Let them know that they are the center of your world and that you would be lost

without them. Compliment your partner. Remind them of the wonderful qualities they have that attracted you to them in the first place. Feeling a mental and emotional closeness to your partner will enhance the physical sensations of making love.

Great Sexpectations

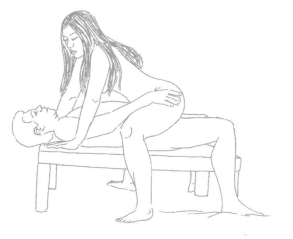

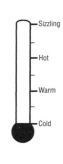

Don't you just love the sexcitement of a great physical sexperience? And you don't need to be a sexpert to sexecute this position. Earn sextra credit points if you orgasm together. So, take a deep breath, sexhale, and get started.

You'll need a coffee table or bench for this position. An ottoman pushed up to the couch works great too. The man lies on his back on the bench with his legs straddling both sides. For the best thrusting, his feet need to be able to reach the ground. The woman sits on top of the man facing him. Her legs are also straddling both sides of the bench.

Ladies, start by sitting on your partner's thighs. Lean forward and let your breasts rub up against his penis. Men find this highly arousing! Using your hand to hold his penis straight, lift your hips and rub the head of your partner's penis against your vulva. They love to be teased! Insert the head of his penis into your vagina, and slowly lower yourself down onto your partner's torso. Lean forward and rub your breasts against his chest. Thrust your hips forward and backward until he reaches his peak.

Self-Indulgence

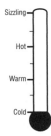

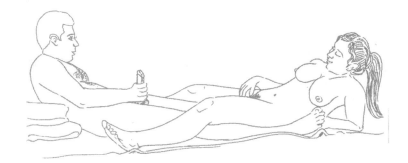

It's hard to say which part is more indulgent: the pleasure of masturbating in front of your partner, or watching your partner masturbate in front of you.

Recline on the bed or floor facing each other. Put one arm behind you to hold your upper body weight. Ladies, to help enhance the closeness of the position, put your legs on top of your partner's legs.

Use your hand and start stimulating your genitals. Make eye contact with each other. Watch your partner while their hands and fingers get them aroused.

Guys, tell your partner what you like and how it feels when you masturbate. Many intercourse positions give you the opportunity to watch your partner masturbate. However, she gets to watch you a lot less

frequently. Talk to her about how it feels to have your hand rubbing up and down your shaft. Show her your most sensitive spots and the best pressure and speed for stimulating them. Describe to her how arousing it is to have her watching you.

Continue indulging yourselves until both of you have climaxed. Then feel free to indulge each other.

Talk the Talk

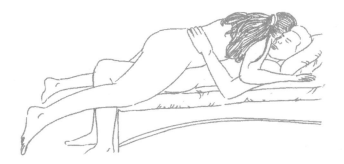

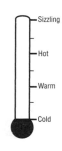

Sizzling

Hot

Warm

Cold

We're not talking about small talk or pillow talk. We're talking about talking dirty. Ladies, this time it's your turn. Decide how racy and raunchy you want to be. Many women find that the dirtier they talk, the more arousing they find the sex. So let yourself go wild.

Have your partner lie on the bed with his legs hanging over the edge. Lean over and tell him that you want his stiff hard cock to be deep inside of you. Put his hands on your breasts while you describe to him how wet and hot and tight you are for him. Describe to him all the things you plan to do to him and all the things you want him to do to you. Be creative. Even if you don't do everything you mention, your partner will find it arousing just hearing you say them.

Stand up and hold his penis in your hand. Ask him if he wants in. When he says yes, tell him you want to suck on him first. Then lower your mouth and make him wet. Look him in the eye as you grab the shaft and slide your hips down onto it. Extend your legs behind you and lean all the way forward so that you are lying on your partner. Spread your legs apart so that your partner's legs are inside your legs.

Grind your hips against your partner each time he thrusts. Describe to him what you're doing as you rub your clitoris back and forth against him. No need to explain your orgasm. Words could never do it justice.

Falling for You

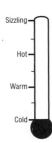

Sizzling —

Hot —

Warm —

Cold —

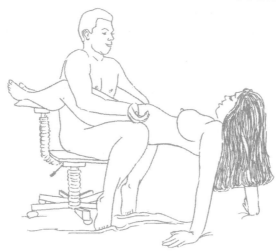

Of all the chair positions in this book, this one has the most unusual angle. Some of you will love it. Others, well, maybe not as much. Give it a try. It might look a little different, but you might just be one of those couples who love it!

Ladies, have your partner sit comfortably on the couch or chair. Sit on his lap facing him. Lean backward a bit and wrap your legs around his chest.

Scoot your bottom forward as far as you can. You want the penetration to be as deep as possible.

Carefully lean all the way backward so that your arms can reach the floor behind you. Make sure you do this slowly. If you rush this step, you're going to hurt your partner, lose penetration, or both. If you do it properly, you'll feel a very tight, although shallow, penetration.

Guys, you will be doing most of the thrusting. Put one hand on your partner's hips to help hold her in place. Use your other hand to manually stimulate her clitoris. Don't drag out your orgasm. This position feels great, but not for an extended period of time. Help your partner back up after both of you have climaxed.

Fire Down Below

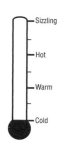

Sizzling

Hot

Warm

Cold

You've felt his fire down below. Sometimes it's just a small flame. At other times, it's raging out of control! This fellatio activity has you fighting fire with fire and making his warmest parts even warmer. Just a word of caution: Be careful when using heat. Your mouth and his genitals are both very sensitive. Hot is good. Burnt is not.

Start by getting a mug of steaming hot liquid. Hold your hands around the mug to get them really warm. Then wrap one hand around your partner's shaft and one hand around his testicles. He'll feel a rush of warmth flow from your hands all through his body. Put some of the hot water in your mouth or hold the mug against your tongue. Lower your mouth around the head of his penis and rub all around it with your hot steamy tongue. Your lover will find the sensations overpowering! Heat your mouth again and take in the head and shaft. Each time you heat up your mouth, the interruption drives your partner crazy with anticipation. After you've done this a few times, your partner will be too aroused to handle any more breaks in the action. Keep your lips sealed around his shaft, lifting and lowering your head until his fire has been extinguished.

Lateral Thinking

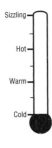

Sizzling

Hot

Warm

Cold

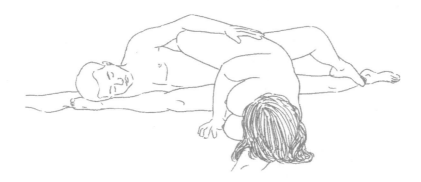

Do you like to think outside the box? Do you pride yourself on solving problems with creative thought and originality rather than traditional conventional thinking? If so, this lateral position will have you thinking about sex in a new and different way.

For this position, the man lies on his side. The woman is also on her side. Her upper body is perpendicular to her partner's body. She has one leg on her partner's chest and one leg draped over his waist.

Guys, you have your partner's foot right next to your face. Put your mouth around her toes and rub your tongue between them. Stroke and caress her leg. Put your hand over her hand as she manually stimulates her clitoris. Time your thrusts so you can orgasm together.

Puck You!

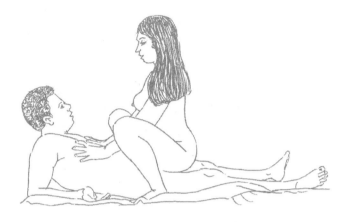

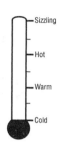

Sizzling

Hot

Warm

Cold

Ladies, check your partner against the boards and grab his stick. We're going to play some hockey and we need to score!

Have your partner lie on his back with his arms behind him and his weight resting on his elbows. Sit on top of your partner's thighs facing him. Your legs should be bent so that your feet are flat on the floor by your partner's hips. Check out his equipment and make sure it meets regulations. It looks like he has some high sticking going on, but there's no need for a penalty. High sticking in this game is good!

Raise your hips and line up your center circle for the face-off. Lower your hips down the shaft of his penis. Slide your hips back and forth on the smooth surface of the rink. While he's taking advantage of the power play inside of you, have your partner rub your clitoris.

He shoots! He scores! Why not go for the hat trick and score twice more!

Tongue Twisters

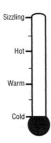

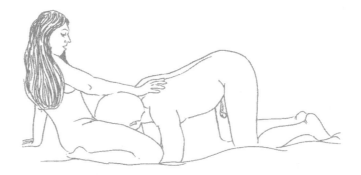

Okay, guys. Try out these tongue twisters to get you ready for this cunnilingus position. If you can say them quickly and correctly three times in a row, you are a tongue-twisting king. And your partner will be one very happy queen!

Harry's Huge Hammer in Hannah's Honey Hole.

Bob's Big Beast Boinking Betty's Big Box.

If you've mastered those, then you are ready to go. Have your partner kneel down with her knees spread apart. You are in front of her on your hands and knees. Put your hands on your partner's hips and lean all the way forward. To get your tongue onto her clitoris, you'll need to bury your face in her pubic hair.

Slide one hand between her legs and use your finger to rub the area around the vagina. Stick your tongue all the way out and rub it against her clitoris. If you're having difficulty getting the angle right, have your partner lean backward. This will make the access a lot easier. Twist your tongue around on her clitoris until she reaches her peak.

Sideshow

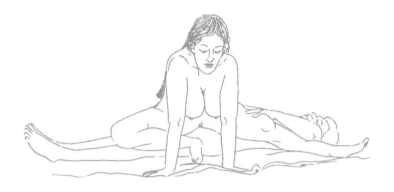

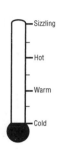

Sizzling

Hot

Warm

Cold

The sideways penetration of this position is definitely the main event! As with all sideways positions, however, lubrication is important. So start with a little sideshow. Guys, use your tongue to make sure your partner is nice and wet. Lick all around the vagina. Stick your tongue inside and lick around the entrance. For this position, wetter is definitely better.

The man lies on his back with his legs together in front of him. Ladies, sit down sideways on top of your partner. With all the lubrication, you should have no difficulty getting his penis to slide inside of you. Bend one leg so that your foot is sideways by your partner's hip. The other leg should be spread open to the side. Lean forward and put your upper body weight on your arms. This will make it much easier to lift and lower your hips and thrust.

Use one hand to stimulate your clitoris. You will probably still feel aroused from the cunnilingus you received from your partner. Thrust your hips and rub your fingers until both of you have climaxed.

Good Vibrations

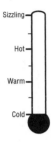

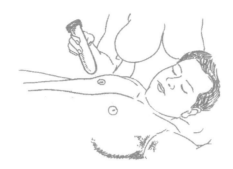

Get out the vibrator, ladies. You'll be using it while you manually stimulate your partner. He is in for a big treat!

Have your partner lie on his back with his legs bent. Sit or kneel between his legs. Turn on the vibrator and rub it over the top of his thighs. Then put some lubrication on the vibrator and let the tip rub up against his anus. Although many men are reluctant to try this activity, the ones that do are overwhelmed at the pleasure they experience. Slowly insert the tip of the vibrator into your partner's anus. You don't need much of the vibrator to penetrate, maybe an inch or so, for the vibrations to cause intense stimulation that your partner will feel from head to foot.

Simultaneously, masturbate his penis with your hand. Stroke the shaft up and down. He'll be begging for you to make him come. Increase the pressure and speed of your stroking until he reaches an orgasmic finish.

The Texas Two-Step

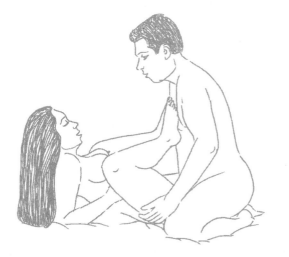

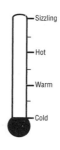

Y'all don't have to live in the Lone Star State to enjoy this position!

The first step is some foreplay. Texas is a hot and dry state. You need to make sure you have an adequate supply of water. Take turns performing oral sex on each other. The goal is not to orgasm, but to arouse each other and get lubricated.

The second step is intercourse. Ladies, lie on your back with your arms behind you so that your head and shoulders are elevated. Bend your legs up to your chest. Guys, kneel down next to your partner with her feet pressed against your chest. Texas is famous for its longhorns, so put your hand around yours

and guide it into your partner's vagina. Lean all the way forward against your partner's feet. This position puts you deep in the heart of Texas. Thrust your hips and continue drilling for oil until your pipeline is overflowing.

Y'all come back and visit this wonderful state as often as you want.

On Bended Knees

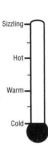

Sizzling

Hot

Warm

Cold

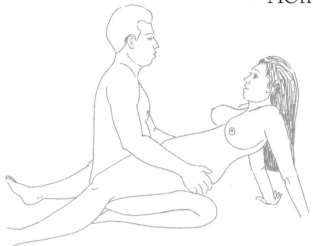

You don't need divine intervention to enjoy this position. All you need is a willing partner!

Ladies, have your partner kneel down so that his legs are completely bent underneath him. Kneel down in front of him and wrap your hand around the shaft of his penis.

Stroke up and down a few times. Tell your partner you're engaging in a little hero worship. It's good for their egos. Guys can be very gullible when it comes to praising their equipment!

Keep your hand on his penis to help guide it inside of you as you sit on your

partner's lap. Spread your legs out wide behind your partner's back. Move your bottom as far forward as you can to get the deepest penetration. Put your arms behind you and lean backward. Let your partner do the thrusting until both of you have had your prayers answered.

Rub You the Right Way

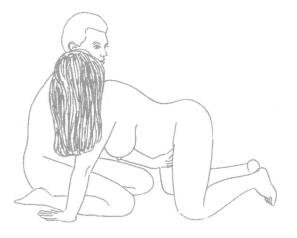

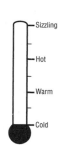

Sizzling

Hot

Warm

Cold

Okay, guys. Here's your chance to make up for all the times you've rubbed her the wrong way and made her mad about something. This position will literally have you rubbing her the right way!

Sit down, cross-legged if you can, on the floor or bed. Have your partner in front of you on her hands and knees. Her head should be by your shoulder.

Slide one hand down between your partner's legs. Gently stroke your fingers all around her vulva. Lightly tap your fingers against her hot, wet skin. Sometimes less can be more, and this is one of those times. Your goal is to get her aroused, interested, and wanting more.

Steadily increase the pressure of your fingertips and start focusing most of your attention on the clitoral area. With your other hand, massage one of her breasts. Tug and tease the nipple. Rub it between your fingers.

Slide your fingers back and forth across your partner's clitoris. You'll feel her start leaning into you when you've found a spot that is particularly stimulating. Continue rubbing it the right way until your partner orgasms.

The Dirty Deed

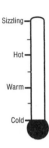

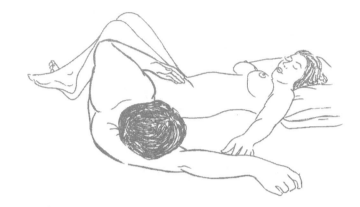

Time to do a little dirty dancing! Guys, if your partner gives you a dirty look when you suggest this position, just remind her that it's a whole lot more fun than washing dirty laundry!

For this position, the man is lying on his side. Ladies, lie on your back with your legs over your partner's hips. In order to achieve penetration, your bottom must be right next to his torso. The closer you can get, the deeper the penetration will be. Penetration will also be improved if you arch your back slightly. For tight penetration, clench your legs together and cross your ankles.

Guys, you will be doing the dirty work. Squeeze your fingers between her legs to stimulate her clitoris as you thrust. With her legs clenched together, there is not a lot of room for your fingers to move around. That's okay. Once your find a sensitive spot, use your fingers to rub the area back and forth. Small, short strokes will do the dirty trick. Continue applying pressure until both of you have peaked.

Head Coach

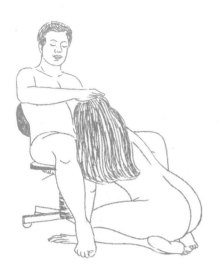

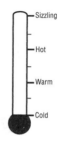

Ladies, you've given enough head that you've earned the right to be the head coach! And, as everyone knows, the head coach gets to call the plays! No need for a whistle, just your tongue.

Have your partner sit in a chair or on the couch. Spread his legs apart and kneel down between them. Start by leaning forward and letting your tongue do a few warm-up stretches on his nipples. Put your mouth around the entire nipple and rub your tongue back and forth. Nipples are a sensitive area for a lot of men and are frequently overlooked.

Bring your head down to his groin and start by licking his testicles. Move your tongue to the base of his shaft and drag it all the way up to the head of his penis. Wrap your lips around the head and let your tongue rub circles all around it. Lower your head further so that at least half of the shaft is covered by your hot mouth. Wrap your hand around the remainder of the shaft. Simultaneously lift and lower your head and hand, being careful to keep at least part of the head in your mouth at all times. A good head coach knows the importance of including the tongue in the game. Have it lick up, down, and all around the penis. Continue the drill until your team is victorious.

Body Chemistry

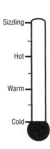

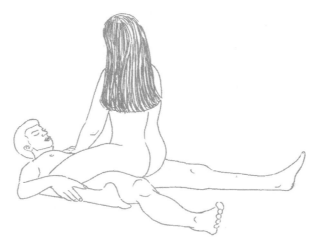

Get out the chemistry set. It's time to establish some covalent molecular bonds with your partner. This experiment is guaranteed to cause an explosive chemical reaction.

Guys, lie on your back with your legs spread apart. Hold your test tube in your hand. Have your partner face you and straddle your torso with her legs bent so that her feet are behind her. Let your test tube slide inside her Bunsen burner. Feel the heat being radiated as you combine your chemical equations.

Ladies, increase the chemical coefficient by stimulating your clitoris with your hand. Feel the surge of kinetic energy being produced. Thrust your hips and rub your fingers until both of you have reached spontaneous combustion.

Split the Difference

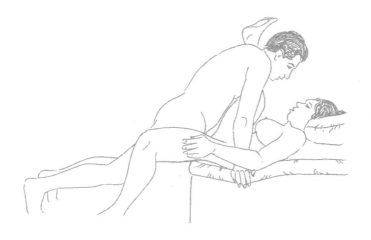

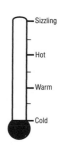

Sizzling

Hot

Warm

Cold

Should her legs be up? Or should her legs be down? Why not split the difference and have one of each!

Ladies, lie on your back with your legs hanging over the edge of the bed. Bring your hips all the way to the edge to enable your partner to penetrate. Leave one leg bent toward the floor. Lift the other leg and put it on your partner's shoulder.

Guys, lean against the bed with your legs straight behind you. Support your upper body weight by placing your arms on the bed in front of you. Have your partner put her hand around your penis to help establish penetration. Adjust the height of your hips, as needed, until you slide inside. Once in, use long, deep thrusts. Pull your hips back so that only a small portion of your penis remains inserted. Then push your hips forward until your entire penis is surrounded by your partner's soft, velvety warmth. Continue thrusting until both of you have peaked.

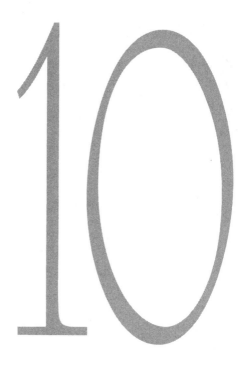

MONTH 10

Day 1. A Close Shave

Day 2. Jigsaw Puzzle

Day 3. Different Strokes . . .

Day 4. Pubic Defender

Day 5. Look Ma, No Hands!

Day 6. Hold Your Tongue

Day 7. Hitting Below the Belt

Day 8. Screw You!

Day 9. The Home Stretch

Day 10. Dressed for

      Success

Day 11. Yin and Yang

Day 12. Step on It

Day 13. Give Her a Hand

Day 14. Love to Love

Day 15. Head Hunter

Day 16. With You by My Side

Day 17. Over and Above

Day 18. On the Rocks

Day 19. Sex Education

Day 20. Plays Well with Self

Day 21. The Naked Truth

Day 22. The Magic Mirror

Day 23. Offer and Honor

Day 24. Musical Chairs

Day 25. Pipe Dreams

Day 26. Kiss and Tell

Day 27. Meat and Potatoes

Day 28. Fooling Around

Day 29. Getting Lucky

Day 30. Main Squeeze

A Close Shave

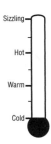

Sizzling

Hot

Warm

Cold

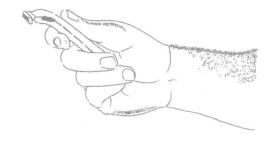

I'm not sure if this is more erotic for the man or the woman. This is an intimate and arousing activity that totally changes the look and feel of sex. Guys, you'll need a pair of scissors, a razor, and some soap or shaving cream. You'll be shaving off your partner's pubic hair.

Have your partner soak in the bathtub for a few minutes to get her skin soft. Then have her sit on a towel on the floor, the bathroom counter, or the side of the bathtub so that her pubic hair is out of the

water. Use the scissors to cut the hair short. This makes it easier when you use the razor and prevents accidentally pulling the pubic hair. (Ouch!) Seductively lather her up with soap or shaving cream. Don't limit yourself to the pubic hair. Soapy hands are smooth and slippery and feel great on the thighs and lower torso too. Carefully use the razor and shave off all the pubic hair. Rinse and dry your partner with a towel. Rub some lotion onto the newly shaved skin to moisturize it.

You will probably be surprised at how different your partner looks and feels. And it doesn't just affect her skin. Your partner will feel aroused and sexy with the new appearance. Use your hands and give her some great manual stimulation. Start by rubbing your hands all around her vulva. Steadily work your way to her clitoris. Encourage your partner to keep one hand on her soft, newly shaved skin while you stimulate her clitoris and bring her to orgasm.

Jigsaw Puzzle

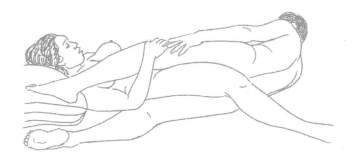

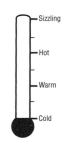

Your interlocking pieces will fit together perfectly with this position.

The male piece of the puzzle needs to be lying on his side. The female piece of the puzzle lies on her back. Ladies, spread your legs apart. Put one leg between your partner's legs and the other leg in front of your partner's chest. Use your hand to guide your partner's penis as you move your hips forward and surround his penis with your warm, wet, silky vagina.

Push your hips forward as far as you can. This makes the penetration deep, but also puts your pubic bone right under your partner's thigh. Maneuver your hips around until you've got a sensitive spot rubbing up against him each time he thrusts. As you start to reach your peak, thrust your hips so that you can get the right pressure and pace. This is stimulating for your partner and will help him reach his climax too.

Different Strokes...

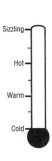

Sizzling
Hot
Warm
Cold

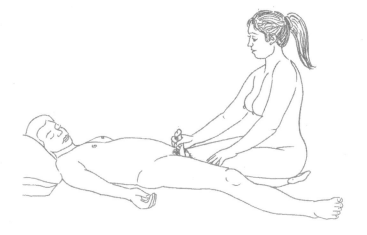

For different folks. Ladies, the key is to try a variety of strokes to help you figure out which kind of stroke your partner likes the most. This manual stimulation position will help you do just that.

Have your partner lie on his back with his legs spread apart. Kneel down between his legs. Make sure your partner gives you feedback on the different types of strokes that you try.

Start with the shaft of your partner's penis between both of your hands. Slide your hands back and forth. You can move both hands in the same direction at the same time, or alternate your hands. While one hand is moving toward you, the other hand is moving away from you. Simultaneously move your hands up and down the shaft.

Many men like a firmer stroke with a more encompassing grip around the shaft. Wrap your hand around the shaft of your partner's penis with your pinky finger at the base and your thumb near the head. Stroke upward from the base to the tip. Quickly turn your hand around for the return stroke. Wrap your hand so that your pinky finger is near the top and your thumb is near the base. Stroke downward from the tip to the base.

Use the stroke that pleases your partner the most. Increase pressure and pace until the finishing stroke has been made.

Pubic Defender

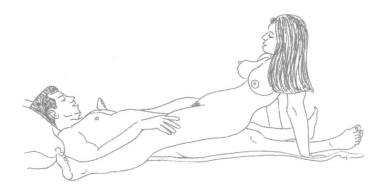

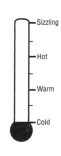

You've been accused of a nasty crime and it's time for your day in court. Although you might be acquitted, the fact that you're reading this book and using this position rules out any innocence.

First you need to find the correct courthouse for the trial. If you're in a location that has witnesses, you'll need a change of venue. These sequestered proceedings will not be part of the public record.

Ladies, summon your partner and have him lie on his back with his legs together. Make sure his briefs have already been filed. Sit on top of him, facing him, with your legs spread apart. Enter his case into your docket as you lower your hips. Put your arms behind you and lean against them.

Have your partner use his hand to stimulate your clitoris until you orgasm. Remind him that if he refuses, he'll be in contempt of court. And don't fake an orgasm. Remember, you're under oath and could get thrown into jail for perjury.

So what's the verdict? This position has met the burden of proof and shown beyond a reasonable doubt that it's fun!

Look Ma, No Hands!

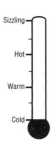

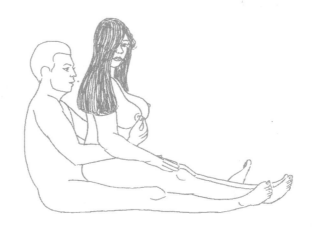

Do you remember how exciting it was when you learned how to ride a bike without holding on? Recapture the moment as you sit in your partner's lap and ride him.

Guys, sit on the floor with your legs out in front of you. Lower your partner onto your lap facing the same direction that you are. Hold your penis steady while she maneuvers her hips and lowers herself down your shaft. For the tightest penetration, your partner's legs should be straight in front of her. If she's not too heavy, have your partner put her legs on top of yours. It increases the amount of skin-to-skin contact.

Wrap your arms around your partner and hold her close. It's such a warm, comfortable feeling to be lovingly embraced during sex. Kiss her ears and neck. Tickle them with your tongue.

Ladies, use your hand to stimulate your clitoris. As your arousal increases, grind your hips into your partner. This is a bicycle built for two. Pace your masturbation so that you and your partner can orgasm together.

Hold Your Tongue

Month 10
Day 6

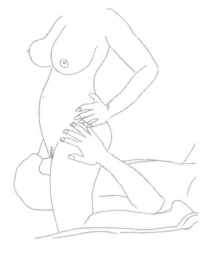

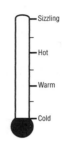

- Sizzling
- Hot
- Warm
- Cold

In fact, hold it right up against your partner. Guys, this is a cunnilingus position that has you lying on your back. Your partner is on her knees straddling your face. She should be facing away from your body. You might need a pillow or two under your head to help you reach all the important spots. It will also help if you hold on to her hips with your hands. It'll save you the aggravation of trying to hit a moving target!

Start by using the tip of your tongue. Use it to gently poke just inside your partner's vagina. She has a lot of nerve endings here and the sensations are very pleasant.

Using short strokes, rub your tongue back and forth across your partner's labia from her vagina to her clitoris. First do it while the labia are together. Then do it again after your tongue has separated them.

Put your mouth around her entire clitoral area. Using just your tongue, pull your partner's clitoral hood aside and expose her clitoris. Rub your tongue back and forth on it. If it's too intense, then put the hood back and continue rubbing with your tongue. Pull your partner's hips down to your face and continue stimulating her until she orgasms.

Hitting Below the Belt

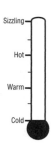

Sizzling —

Hot —

Warm —

Cold —

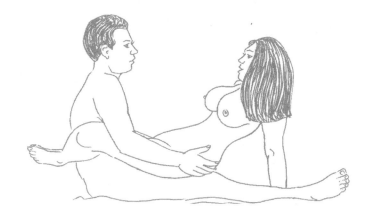

The woman's legs around the man's waist in this position make a belt that will be a big hit below his belt.

The man sits on the bed or floor with his legs spread apart. Ladies, give your partner a low blow. Lean forward between his legs and wrap your mouth around his penis. Make sure he's completely hard, wet, and ready for you to sit on his lap. Wrap your legs around his waist and cross your ankles behind his back. Push your hips all the way forward so that your vulva keeps hitting him below the belt. Put your arms behind you and lean backward.

Guys, be a true and fair sportsman and use your hands to massage your partner above the belt. Caress her breasts. Stroke her sides. As you approach your peak, grab your partner's hips and pull her all the way to you. This will make for a deep and powerful orgasm.

In the 1860s the Marquis of Queensberry rules banned hitting below the belt in boxing. Thankfully, *this* hitting-below-the-belt position is still legal.

Screw You!

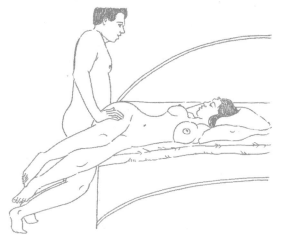

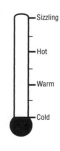

You'd have to have a screw loose not to love this position!

Ladies, sit against the side of the bed with your partner standing in front of you. Take a look at your partner's hardware. You need to make sure his head is screwed on right.

Keep your legs over the side of the bed and lie backward. Your partner should stand next to the bed with his legs bent so that his knees and thighs are pressed up against the side of the bed. Corkscrew your hips to the side so that both of your legs are to the same side of your partner's legs. Lower your hips as far over the edge of the bed as you can to make penetration easier for your partner. Reach your hand behind you and wrap it around your partner's testicles. Fondle them between your fingers.

Guys, don't be a screwup. It's time to put the screws to your partner. Thrust your hips forward so you're in nice and deep. Use your hand to manually stimulate your partner's clitoris. The more fun it is to screw around, the more frequently both of you will get to do this!

The Home Stretch

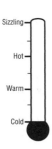

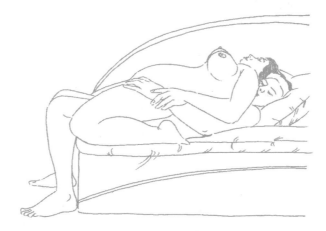

You don't need to stretch your imagination to find things to like about this position. It's deep, intimate, and a lot of fun!

The man lies on his back with his legs over the edge of the bed. Ladies, start out by sitting on your partner's lap facing away from him. Your legs should be bent so that your feet are behind you. Once you've got your partner's penis snug inside of you, lean backward until you are completely lying on your partner. You can't do much thrusting, but you can feel your partner thrusting deep inside of you.

Guys, I don't think you need much help figuring out what to do with this one. You've got two free hands and your partner lying on your chest! Wrap your arms around her and massage her breasts. When she lies on her back, her breasts flatten out toward her sides. Place your hands on the outsides of the breasts to feel their fullness. Stroke the nipples with just your thumbs. As you get to the home stretch, wrap your arms around your partner and hold her tight. Tell her you love her and then climax.

Dressed for Success

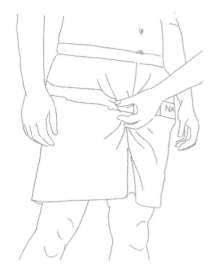

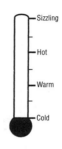

Guys hate to admit it, but generally speaking, they're pretty easy. So, ladies, your goal with this activity is to make your partner orgasm without even unzipping his pants.

Assuming you're not in a public place, and he's not wearing expensive pants, start by blowing on him through his pants. Put your mouth next to the fabric and exhale hard enough to force your hot breath through the material. This is a great tease! Your mouth is in the right area and he can feel the heat, but it's not wet and there's no tongue.

You should be able to feel the shaft of your partner's penis under his pants. Use your hand to stroke up and down it a few times. When men get erect with their pants on, their penis does not always end up hanging at a comfortable angle. It's always nice if you can reach inside of his pants and straighten him out. He'll be most appreciative of this. Resume stroking his penis through his pants. Simultaneously kiss him on the ears, neck, and lips. Continue rubbing your hand along his pants until he reaches his peak.

Yin and Yang

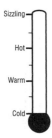

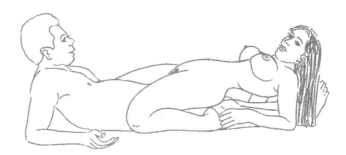

Yin and yang, basic principles of traditional Chinese cosmology, represent feminine and masculine powers or forces. Yin, the female component, is associated with the earth and darkness. The male element, yang, is associated with heaven and light.

Guys, lay your heavenly body down on the bed with your arms behind you and your weight resting on your elbows. The earth is about to enter into your orbit. Ladies, straddle your partner, facing him, with your legs bent so that your feet are behind you. Have your partner guide his radiant light into the deepest, blackest depths of your darkness. Lean backward, bending your arms behind you so that you can rest your weight on your elbows.

Guys, since you're the active and strong force, you should be responsible for manually stimulating your partner. Support your weight on one arm and use your other hand to rub your partner's clitoris. Feel the positive flow of energy as both of you reach your peak.

Step on It

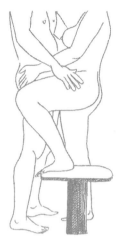

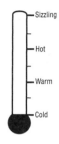

Sizzling

Hot

Warm

Cold

This is a standing position that has the couple facing each other, instead of the usual standing rear-entry pose.

The difficulty with this position is in achieving penetration. The woman should stand on her tiptoes with her legs spread slightly apart. The man's legs should be spread apart a little wider than the woman's legs. His knees should be bent so that he can get the tip of his penis lined up with his partner's vagina. Penetration will occur when the woman lowers herself back onto flat feet and the man raises himself by straightening his legs. To make the position deeper and the thrusting easier, the woman should lift one foot up onto a stool or bathtub.

Put your arms around your partner and hold each other close. Let your chests rub together while you stroke each other's back. Snuggle your faces up next to each other. Kiss and talk quietly together. Make eye contact and let your partner know how happy you are to be there with them. You'll feel an emotional high in addition to the physical high when you orgasm.

Give Her a Hand

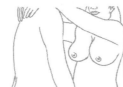
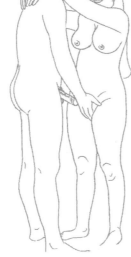

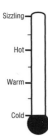

And she knows exactly where she wants you to put it! Guys, this is a position where you will be manually stimulating your partner. So limber up your fingers and get started.

Stand in front of your partner, facing her. Start by holding her close and giving her a tight hug. Kiss her on the lips. Start with soft gentle kisses. Open your lips and wait for her tongue to come looking for yours. Hugging and kissing are elements of love and sex that are easy to take for granted.

Continue standing close enough to your partner that you can rub between her legs with the head of your penis. Many women find this erotic, and it's certainly stimulating for you too. As her arousal increases, switch over to using your fingers. They are much more adept at finding the hot spots! Rub circles around her clitoris. Feel her hips pushing up against your hand. When you find a great spot, rub it back and forth. Let your partner hold on tight as you bring her to orgasm.

Ladies, don't forget to give your partner a hand for giving you a hand.

Love to Love

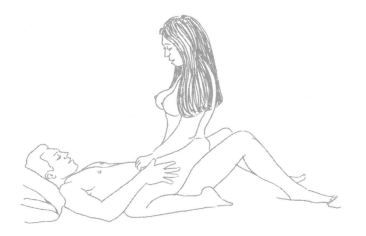

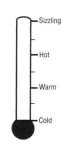

Sizzling

Hot

Warm

Cold

Ladies, it's your serve. Lay your partner on his back with his legs bent at the knees. Sit on his thighs, facing him, with your legs bent so that your feet are behind you. Practice a few of your strokes. Forehand and backhand shots are good, but the overhead shot is the best. Rub your hand all over the head of his racket.

Lift your hips and position yourself over your partner's penis. Serve your partner an ace as you slide your net over his racket. Reach behind you and wrap your hand around his testicles. Volleying his balls is good. Lobbing them over his head is not.

Thrust your hips back and forth. Maintain a steady rhythm and pace. You don't want to make any unforced errors. As the game nears an end, put your fingers around the base of his penis. This is an approach shot that is sure to win you points.

Why stop at just one game? Why not go for game, set, and match?

Head Hunter

Sizzling

Hot

Warm

Cold

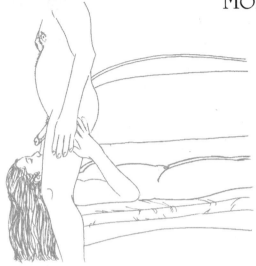

Looking for a blow job? Then it's time to visit a head hunter!

Ladies, lie on your back with your head at the edge of the bed. Depending on the height of your partner, you'll probably need to put a pillow or two under your neck so you can reach him better. Have your partner straddle your face facing away from the rest of your body.

Reach your arm around your partner and wrap your hand around the shaft of his penis. This will give you some control over how deep you want his penis to be inside of your mouth. Start by putting your mouth around just the head. Pull it in and out of your mouth while you suck it.

Allow the shaft of your partner's penis to enter your mouth. Let him thrust his hips, moving the penis in and out. Flick your tongue all around the shaft with each stroke. Your partner gets a great view of his penis as it slides into and out of your mouth. To say he'll find this arousing is an understatement! Continue head hunting until the job has been finished.

Remember: Head hunters work on commission. Have your partner pay your fee by satisfying you!

With You by My Side

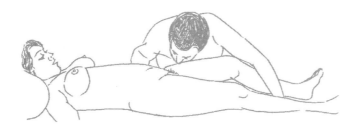

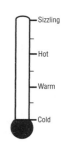

Guys, this is a cunnilingus position where you are sitting or kneeling next to your partner. It changes the angle of your tongue and also gives you lots of opportunities for additional stimulation.

Have your partner lie on her back with her legs spread apart. Lean over and lick her nipples. Alternate your attention between your partner's two breasts. If her breasts are large enough, push them together with your hands and dart your tongue back and forth between the nipples.

Kiss your partner from her breasts down to the tops of her thighs. Use your tongue to lightly tickle her labia. At the same time, use one finger to lightly stimulate the area around the vagina. Insert your finger about an inch and rub it against the inside of the vaginal entrance. Try different amounts of pressure to determine what your partner likes the most.

At the same time, use your tongue to spread apart her labia. Lick the area all around the clitoris. Since you're at a side angle, it's a little more difficult to latch your mouth completely over her clitoris. So stimulate the clitoris by flattening your tongue and covering the entire area with a back-and-forth motion. Watch your partner's responses to find a pressure and pace that will bring her to orgasm.

Over and Above

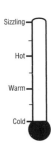

Sizzling

Hot

Warm

Cold

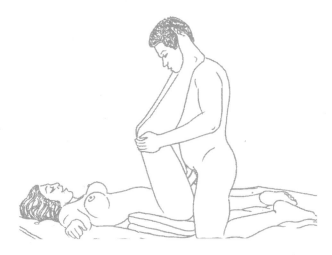

With your legs over his shoulders and his face above yours, this position gives you pleasure over and above what you can get from other positions.

The woman lies on her back. Place a pillow or two under your hips to elevate them. This will make penetration a lot easier. Guys, you are kneeling between your partner's legs. Put her legs in front of you so that she can rest her calves on your shoulders. Have your partner help you line up your penis so that when you thrust your hips you'll smoothly slide inside of her. Lean your weight forward and rest it on your arms.

Because your partner's legs are up on your shoulders, this is a very deep position. The further you lean forward, the deeper it will be. Press your partner's legs as close to her chest as you can without causing her discomfort.

Ladies, give your partner a hug with your legs. Men love to feel your soft, smooth skin next to their neck and face. Clench your vaginal muscles at the same time. It's the small details like these that turn good sex into great sex!

On the Rocks

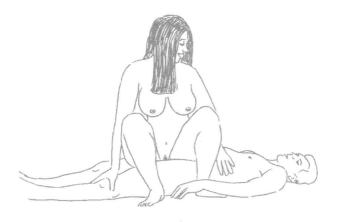

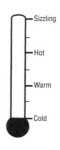

Hope this describes your drink and not your relationship!

For this position, the man lies on his back with his legs straight in front of him. Ladies, you will be sitting sideways on your partner. Your legs should be bent so that your feet are flat on the bed next to him. Spread your knees apart for maximum depth in penetration.

Reach down between your partner's legs and fondle his testicles with your fingers. This will definitely help him get his rocks off. Use your other hand to hold a vibrator and use it to masturbate. Remember, the intensity of the vibrator makes many women orgasm faster than when they just use their fingers. So if you want to climax at the same time as your partner, you might want to start out slowly and simply rub the vibrator in your pubic hair and along the tops of your thighs. As your partner's arousal increases, move the vibrator to your clitoris for maximum pleasure.

Sex Education

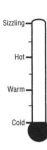

Sizzling

Hot

Warm

Cold

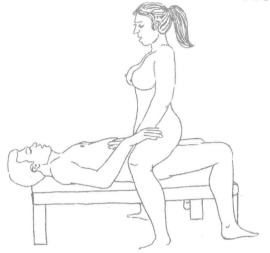

You don't want to be absent for this class! In fact, this is night school and staying for detention would actually be fun. Unlike most schools, however, this class is taught on the desk, not at it.

Ladies, you're the teacher. Have your pupil lie on your desk with his legs straddling the sides. Lean over next to your partner and wrap your mouth around his penis. Head of the class just took on a whole new meaning!

Straddle your partner, facing him. Lower your hips, letting his ruler slide into your pencil box. Put his hand on your clitoris and give him a lesson on manual stimulation. A good student will see the beauty of his partner's great learning curves. And, if he's a quick learner, he'll move your hand aside and take over the demonstration. Both you and your partner can help with the thrusting with this position. If you time things right, you both should hear school bells ringing.

Plays Well with Self

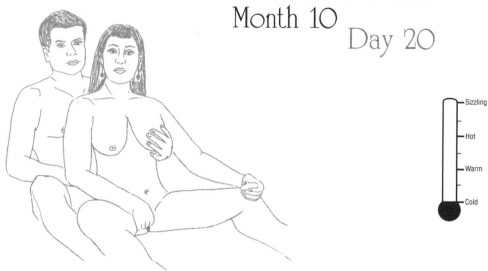

Sizzling

Hot

Warm

Cold

This is a loving and intimate position that has each of you masturbating. Sit down with the woman in front of the man. Both of you should have your legs spread open.

Ladies first tonight. Lean backward against your partner's chest. Put your hand between your legs to stimulate your clitoris. Guys, put your arms around your partner and massage her breasts. Kiss her neck and ears. Tell her how wonderful she is and how much you love to be with her. Hold her tight as she brings herself to her peak.

And, guys, now it's your turn. Pull your partner close enough to you so that you can rub the head of your penis against her skin as you stroke. Ladies, rub your hands along your partner's thighs. Scratch his legs lightly with your fingernails. Gently pull the hair on his legs. Some men find that a small amount of pain enhances their pleasure. Lean into your partner until he reaches his orgasm.

The Naked Truth

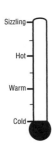

Sizzling

Hot

Warm

Cold

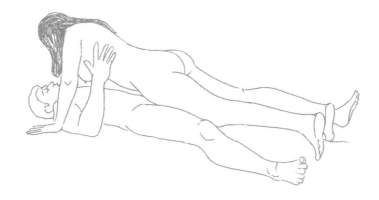

Strip down to your birthday suit. You've got to be in the buff to get the bare facts about this position.

This is a very intimate woman-on-top position with lots of skin contact. So, guys, lie down on your back with your legs spread apart. Ladies, you'll be lying down on top of your partner. The easiest way to get there is to start out by sitting on him with your legs bent so that your feet are behind you. Have your partner hold his penis while you slide your hips down over him. Lean forward so that your weight is on your arms and extend your legs together behind you. Finally, lean all the way forward so that your breasts are rubbing on your partner's chest.

Guys, put your arms around your partner. Stroke her back and sides.

Put one hand behind your partner's head and lower her face so you can kiss her. Let your partner decide how deep she wants the kisses to be. Some women like lots of tongue while others prefer a softer, shallower kiss. Encourage your partner to rock her hips until both of you have a chance to orgasm.

The Magic Mirror

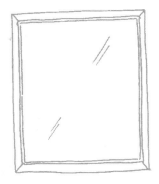

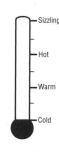

Ladies, if you've never had a chance to watch your partner's penis in your vagina, you're in for a very erotic treat. Because of the design of the female anatomy, it's difficult for women to view intercourse as it's occurring. Men, however, do this regularly and find it stimulating. Just ask your partner if you're not convinced.

The easiest way for a woman to accomplish this is to watch intercourse in a mirror. For the best view, place a large mirror on the floor or bed and use the standard doggy-style position. Get on your hands and knees, straddling the mirror so that you can see your entire vulva. Look in the mirror while your partner guides his penis to your vagina. Pay particular attention as your vagina expands around the head of his penis. Watch as his entire shaft slides deep inside of you.

Use your hand to manually stimulate your clitoris. Look in the mirror as you do this. Continue watching until both of you have reached your peaks.

Offer and Honor

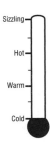

Sizzling

Hot

Warm

Cold

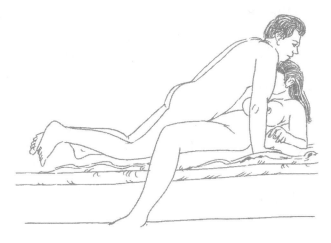

She offers her honor. He honors her offer.

Guys, have your partner lie on her back with her arms bent behind her and her weight on her elbows. She should be next to the edge of the bed so that one leg can be hanging off the side and one leg is straight in front of her.

Lie between your partner's legs with your upper body weight on your arms in front of you, and your legs extended behind you. Maneuver your hips so that the head of your penis just enters your partner's vagina. Thrust your hips forward and let your penis slide deep inside of her.

Rub your chest up against her breasts. Brush her nipples with your chest hairs. Encourage your partner to thrust her hips. With her leg hanging over the side of the bed, she should be able to use her foot to push up off the floor. Synchronize your thrusting with hers until you reach your peak.

Then, of course, you need to get off her. Feel free to continue the pattern all night. On her. Off her. On her. Off her. Honor. Offer.

Musical Chairs

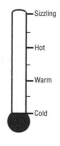

Sizzling

Hot

Warm

Cold

You know the rules for musical chairs. You should always have one chair fewer than the number of people playing the game. Since there are two of you playing, that means you only need one chair. Ladies, my advice is to make sure your partner wins and gets the seat when the music stops. Of course, since you get to sit on his lap, you get to be a winner too!

Once your partner is seated comfortably in his chair, play a little mouth music on his penis. You want to get him hard, slippery, and eager for you. Then sit on his lap, facing him. Your legs should be straddling his lap and hanging down toward the floor. Your partner might have to move his bottom closer to the edge of the chair to enable your legs to hang down at the sides.

After he's inside of you, place your partner's hands on your breasts. Put your hands over his hands and show him how you like to have your breasts massaged. Rub his palms across your nipples. Place his fingers around your nipples and show him how much pressure you'd like him to use. It feels nice for you, plus it's very erotic (and educational) for your partner. Thrust your hips along his instrument until both of you have finished making music.

Pipe Dreams

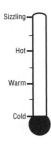

Sizzling
Hot
Warm
Cold

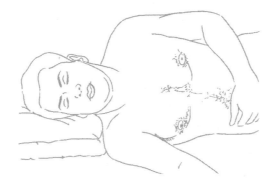

Ladies, you'll have to wait until your partner is sleeping to start this fellatio activity. But, as soon as you put your mouth around his pipe, he'll be having very pleasant dreams.

Hopefully, your partner is sleeping on his back or side. If he's on his stomach, you'll need to pull the covers and gently prod him until he rolls over. Get into a position where your mouth has access to your partner's penis and wrap your lips around it. Regardless of whether he's already erect

or not, put the head and as much of the shaft as you can into your mouth and rub around on it with your tongue. If he wasn't erect when you started, he'll get erect pretty quickly. Fondle your partner's testicles with your fingers while you lick all around the head and shaft of his penis.

Although most men will get erect and moan in pleasure while they're sleeping, very few will actually stay asleep during the orgasm. Part of the fun of this position is the

intense rush your partner gets when he wakes up totally aroused, especially if his penis is still in your mouth. So, if your partner is a deep sleeper and it looks like he might actually sleep through this whole activity, wake him up before he climaxes. Not only will he feel the overwhelmingly pleasant sensations, he'll actually remember it all the next morning. It wasn't just a nighttime pipe dream. It was a dream come true.

Kiss and Tell

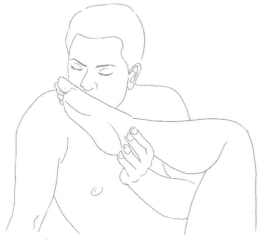

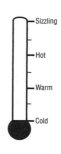

Sizzling

Hot

Warm

Cold

Guys, this is a very romantic cunnilingus activity. You do lots of kissing and your partner tells you how great you are!

Start with your partner's feet. Kiss the sole of her foot from her heel to her toes, paying particular attention to the very sensitive arch. Put each toe into your mouth and suck on it. Kiss all around your partner's ankle. Lovingly caress your partner's calves with your fingers and tongue. Make it your

mission to find and stimulate the most erogenous, most neglected spots on her legs.

Delicately kiss the soft skin at the top of your partner's thighs. Brush your lips against her labia, barely touching them. Tease her by lightly licking around her vagina. You want your partner to be begging you for more! Increase the pressure of your tongue as you rub it against her vagina. Point your tongue and drag it upward between

her labia. Plant a kiss directly onto your partner's clitoris. Using just your lips, gently suck on her clitoris. Then rub your tongue back and forth across her clitoris to bring her to a happy ending.

Ladies, you're responsible for the telling half of this kiss-and-tell activity. Be sure to lavish your partner with encouragement and praise. It'll make him want to do this activity frequently!

Meat and Potatoes

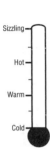

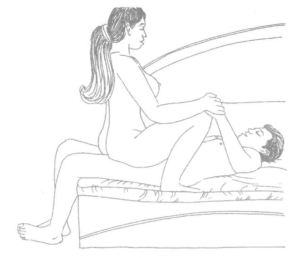

Ladies, get ready for some fresh, juicy meat. And, for those of you that are vegetarians, just pretend we're talking about tofu.

Have your partner lie on his back with his legs hanging over the edge of the bed. Lean over and inspect his meat. A thorough inspection requires sampling the meat for taste. Wrap your lips around your partner's penis and let your mouth water.

Sit on top of your partner, facing him, with your legs bent and your feet flat on the bed next to his hips. Use your hand to guide your partner's meat into your vagina. Clench your vaginal muscles to make this an extra tight position.

Reach down behind you and wrap your hand around your partner's potatoes. Good potatoes always complement great meat. Fondle and stroke them lightly with your fingers. We don't need them mashed! Lift and lower yourself along your partner's shaft until he's finished making gravy.

Fooling Around

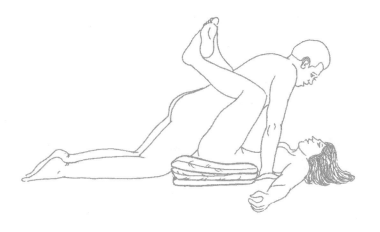

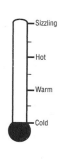

You'd have to be a fool not to love having your partner's legs around your waist in this position! So stick around. There's plenty to go around.

This position is a variation of the standard missionary position. The woman lies on her back with a pillow or two under her hips to elevate them. This minor modification makes this variation much deeper than the standard missionary position. The man leans forward between the woman's legs with his legs straight behind him. After he's achieved penetration, the woman should wrap her legs around her partner's waist.

Ladies, use your legs to pull your partner close to you. He'll know you're serious, and not just messing around. Stroke his face, hair, and neck. Rub his nipples with your fingers and make them taut. Men love it when they get extra attention from their lover. Lift your hips to meet your partner's as he thrusts. Prove the adage that what goes around will come around.

Getting Lucky

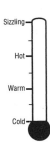

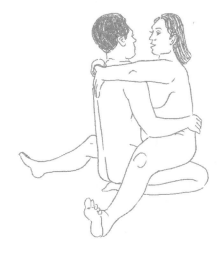

Feeling lucky tonight? Well, you've just gotten a lucky break. So, thank your lucky stars, grab your good luck charm, and get ready to get lucky.

For this position, the man kneels with his legs completely bent underneath him. Ladies, you will be sitting on your partner's lap with your legs spread out wide behind him. Start by just teasing him. Let the tip of his penis rub against your vulva. Insert the head and slowly slide your hips about halfway down the shaft of your partner's penis. After a few shallow thrusts, lower yourself all the way down to your partner's lap. You want to feel him deep inside of you, and he wants to feel that too!

Guys, hold your partner close and let her breasts rub against your chest. Kiss her gently and lovingly tickle her neck. As you approach your orgasm, let her know that you're the luckiest man alive to have her as a partner.

Main Squeeze

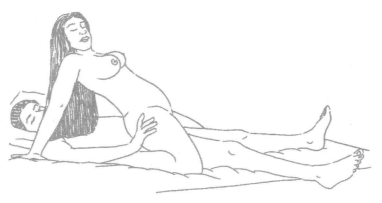

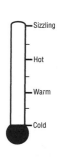

Sizzling

Hot

Warm

Cold

Get your main squeeze, go into the bedroom, and run a squeeze play!

The man lies on his back with his legs spread open wide. Ladies, straddle your partner on his torso facing his feet. Your legs should be bent so that your feet are behind you. Squeeze your thighs together around his penis. Let your partner feel how hot and wet you are for him.

Lift your hips and lower yourself onto your partner's penis. Put your arms behind you and lean backward. If your hair is long enough, lower your head behind you and drag your hair across your partner's chest, as you put one hand between your legs and stimulate your clitoris. Squeeze your vaginal muscles together as you and your main squeeze reach your peaks.

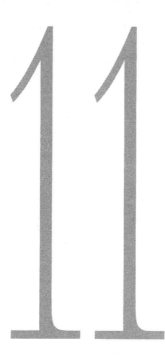

MONTH 11

Day 1. The Nasty Habit

Day 2. With Open Arms

Day 3. Assets Under Management

Day 4. Follow the Bouncing Ball

Day 5. Wet and Wild

Day 6. Organ Donor

Day 7. The Doctor Is In

Day 8. Brain Teaser

Day 9. Mission Not Impossible

Day 10. Touch and Go

Day 11. What's Cooking

Day 12. Royally Screwed

Day 13. Hold Your Fire

Day 14. Get Over It!

Day 15. The Love God

Day 16. A Sticky Situation

Day 17. Love Seat

Day 18. Wrong-Hand Man

Day 19. Hot Under the Collar

Day 20. Birds of a Feather . . .

Day 21. Horsing Around

Day 22. Man in the Moon

Day 23. Hot and Tasty

Day 24. Straddle the Fence

Day 25. Double Cross

Day 26. Vibrator Madness

Day 27. Face Value

Day 28. Gone Fishing

Day 29. Holding the Torch

Day 30. It Takes Two

The Nasty Habit

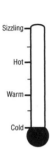

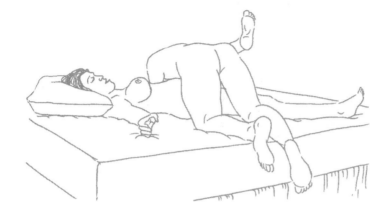

That you don't want to break! If anything, your resolution should be to indulge in this habit more often.

This position has you doing the nasty with sideways penetration. The woman lies on her back. The man lies on top of the woman at a 90 degree angle to her. You might find it difficult to establish penetration when starting from the sideways angle. If so, start in the standard missionary position and rotate around, on your arms, to the side.

Ladies, wrap one of your legs around your partner's waist. Use it to pull your partner down to you so he can be inside of you as deep as possible. Maneuver your hips until your partner bumps up against a sensitive spot on you each time he thrusts. Use your hands to massage your partner's buttocks. Inform him that he has been nasty and naughty, and give him a spanking. Some men like it hard enough to cause pain; others don't want any pain at all. Experiment until you find out exactly what your partner likes.

Give up some other habit. And make a habit of using this position regularly.

With Open Arms

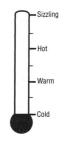

Sizzling

Hot

Warm

Cold

Ladies, I don't think you'll need to twist your partner's arm to stand in front of you and enjoy this manual stimulation position. So, don't keep him at arm's length. Pull your partner close until you're wrapped around him like a coat of arms.

Rub your hands on your partner's chest. Tickle his nipples. Slide your hands down your partner's stomach until you reach his groin. Brush your hand up against his penis and then bring both hands back up to his chest. Your partner is waiting for you to wrap your hand around his penis, but make him wait a little longer. Tease him a few more times by rubbing his chest, dragging your fingers down his stomach, lightly stroking his penis, and then returning your hands to his chest. This builds the anticipation and intensifies the rush he feels when you finally give in to his desires.

Use both of your hands to stimulate your partner. Wrap one hand around the shaft and use the other to stroke the head. Rub the head against the palm of your hand. Run all of your fingers along the edge of the head. Gently pull them up and off the tip. These movements by themselves are probably not enough to make your partner orgasm, but they certainly contribute to the overall experience. Stroke the shaft with the other hand. Use a firm grip that generates lots of friction. Continue stroking, increasing the speed if that's what your partner likes, until he reaches his peak.

Ass-ets Under Management

Month 11
Day 3

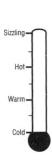

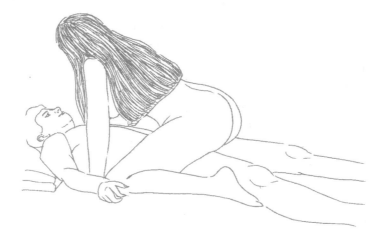

It's time to exercise some fiscal responsibility. As always, read the prospectus before you start investing. Don't send a proxy. You're the primary stockholder for this exchange.

Ladies, have your partner lie on his back with his legs spread open wide. Sit on top of your partner's thighs, facing him, with your legs bent so that your feet are behind you. Tease him a bit by gently rubbing your hand along the shaft of his penis.

Put your hand between your legs and be sure you've got enough liquid assets for this transaction. Raise your hips and add your partner's stock to your portfolio. Lean all the way forward toward your partner. Not only does this make the penetration deeper, it also lets you rub your breasts into your partner's chest.

Thrust your hips up and down, building equity. With good market timing, both of you will see a simultaneous return on your investment. No need to reinvest your partner's deposit. New dividends will be paid with each transaction.

Follow the Bouncing Ball

Month 11
Day 4

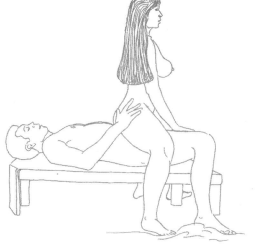

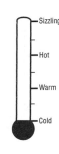

- Sizzling
- Hot
- Warm
- Cold

Get the ball rolling by finding the right spot to engage in this position. Both the man and woman will be straddling a piece of furniture. A table, bench, or an ottoman pushed up to the couch will work. Ideally, the man should be able to reach the floor with his feet.

The man lies on his back with one leg on each side of the bench. The woman sits on top of the man facing his feet. She should also have one leg on each side of the bench.

Ladies, gently grab your partner by the testicles. Remember that you are supposed to be pleasantly stimulating him, not breaking his balls. Fondle them between your fingers. Wrap your hand around them and gently squeeze.

Ask your partner to stroke your back and sides. Encourage him to massage your hips and buttocks.

Don't drop the ball on taking care of yourself. Place your hand between your legs and manually stimulate your clitoris. Thrust your hips and masturbate until both of you have had a ball!

Wet and Wild

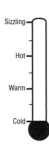

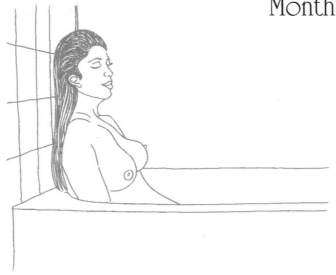

This underwater cunnilingus activity certainly qualifies as both! Guys, have your partner get into a bathtub full of warm, soapy water. Start by lathering up your partner's upper body and legs. Rub her all over with your soapy hands.

Spread your partner's legs apart and touch her vulva with your fingers. Her labia will be soft, and maybe a bit swollen, from the water. The easiest way to perform cunnilingus on your partner is to get into the bathtub with her, on your knees between her legs. This allows you to put your hands under her buttocks and lift her hips up out of the water. The goal is to move her clitoris closer to the surface of the water, but without raising it out of the water completely.

Lower your mouth into the water and rub your tongue back and forth across your partner's clitoris. You'll notice that cunnilingus feels different when your tongue is underwater. Your partner will feel smooth and slippery. Your tongue slides back and forth easily. Find the spots that your partner finds the most arousing and continue stimulating them with your tongue. Don't stop until your partner has made a big splash!

Organus Donor

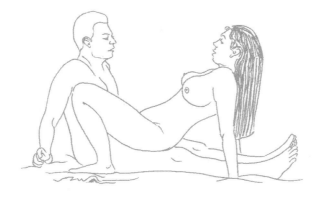

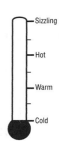

There is only one organ we're talking about here and you're not donating it to science. Guys, get yourself organ-ized so you can transplant your organ deep inside your partner.

For this position, the organ donor sits on the bed with his legs out straight in front of him. Transplants work best when the organ is hot and stiff.

The organ recipient sits on the lap of the organ donor, facing him. Her legs should be bent so that her feet are flat on the floor next to the donor's hips. Once the transplant is complete and the donor's organ slides smoothly inside the recipient, she should put her arms behind her and lean backward.

Guys, use your hands to massage your partner's breasts and stimulate her clitoris. Let her vulva press into your hand each time your partner thrusts her hips. Keep your organ inside your partner until it has made its final donation.

The Doctor Is In

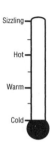

Sizzling

Hot

Warm

Cold

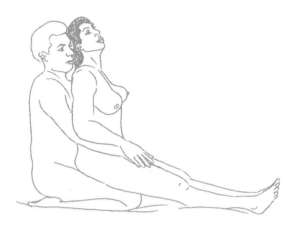

Is there a doctor in the house? I hope so because we have a serious case that needs to be diagnosed and treated immediately. An examination of your symptoms reveals that you and your partner are suffering from a chronic case of sexualitis. This is extremely contagious and should be taken care of immediately.

For this position, the doctor is kneeling on the bed or floor with his legs completely bent underneath him. Ladies, you are the head nurse and you need to make sure your partner has plenty of fluids. Lean over and wrap your mouth around his penis. It's the head nurse's job to get his head and shaft prepped for surgery.

Guys, have your partner sit down on your lap facing the same direction that you are facing. Her legs should be straight in front of her. Check your partner's vital signs. As arousal and stimulation increase, her blood pressure will rise, her pulse will quicken, her respiration will become rapid and shallow, and she will probably feel very warm and feverish.

The best known cure for this condition is to continue thrusting until all signs of the ailment have been ejaculated and the nervous system has returned to normal. To help induce recurrences, I prescribe a daily dose of great sex.

Brain Teaser

Sizzling

Hot

Warm

Cold

Did you ever notice that when men get aroused they quit thinking with the head on their shoulders? Well, this fellatio position teases and tantalizes the brain in the lower head.

Ladies, lie on your back. Have your partner get on his knees and straddle your face. He should be facing away from the rest of your body. Wrap your hand around the shaft of your partner's penis to give you better control.

Lick all around the head of your partner's penis. Don't put the head in your mouth. Instead, just drag your tongue all around it. This is definitely a tease, and guys love it!

Insert just the head of your partner's penis into your mouth. Now lick all around the head from inside of your hot, wet mouth. Rub your tongue along the slit on the underside of the head. Your partner is going to try

and thrust some of his shaft into your mouth too. Keep your hand in place on the shaft until you decide you've teased him enough and you're ready to move on.

Let your partner thrust his penis into your sweet mouth. Rub your tongue up and down the shaft as it slides in and out. Your partner should continue thrusting until he's brain dead.

Mission Not Impossible

Month 11
Day 9

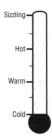

Sizzling

Hot

Warm

Cold

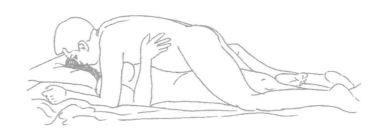

Your mission, if you should choose to accept it, is to have great sex today, and every day. Doesn't sound like a very difficult mission to me!

Today's position will help you get started toward your goal. The woman is on her back on the bottom. The man is on top in a traditional missionary pose with his legs straight out behind him. The difference between this position and the regular missionary position is that the man and woman have their legs entwined. The man has one leg between the woman's legs, and the woman has one leg between the man's legs. This subtle difference causes the position to be more romantic, but also much more shallow. So, ladies, clench your vaginal muscles to maximize the amount of friction being generated.

You're pretty much set up for good sex, but we're looking for great sex. One of the biggest benefits of this position is the intimacy created by being face-to-face with your partner. Look your partner in the eyes and really see them. Stroke their face. Smile at them. Often couples see each other every day, but don't really see each other at all. Truly connect with your partner before, during, and after your orgasm.

Touch and Go

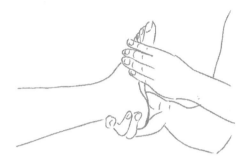

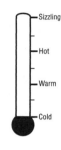

Sizzling

Hot

Warm

Cold

This is a massage activity that finishes when the man manually stimulates his partner's clitoris. The other massage activities in this book have the person being massaged lying on their back. For men, it's only practical. After all, it's hard to stroke a man's penis when he's lying on his stomach. But for women, this is not necessarily true. A woman can have her clitoris stimulated even when she's on her tummy.

So, guys, have your partner lie face down on the bed or carpet. Start by giving her a neck and shoulder rub. Use your fingers to relax the muscles and release her tension. Work your way down her back using long sweeping motions with the full hand. Spread your fingers apart to cover the maximum surface area you are massaging. Place your outstretched hands on your partner's back and pull your fingers to the center, pushing down gently with them as you do this.

Caress your partner's buttocks. Knead the soft fleshy skin between your thumbs and fingers. Put a hand on each cheek and firmly massage it with your fingers. Work one hand between her legs and caress the tops of her inner thighs. Steadily work your way to your partner's clitoral area. You don't have much room, but you should be able to work your fingers back and forth across her clitoris. Feel as she pushes her vulva into your hand as she reaches her peak.

What's Cooking

Sizzling—

Hot—

Warm—

Cold—

Turn up the heat! It looks like we're cooking a rump roast!

This is a great rear-entry position where the woman leans against a kitchen counter. Of course, a bathroom counter or dresser will work too. But I think the kitchen is the best place for cooking meat.

Ladies, stand in front of your partner facing the same direction he is. Spread your legs apart and lean forward against the counter. Use your hand, with an oven mitt around it if your partner is really hot, and guide your partner's meat into your oven. Push your hips backward as your partner thrusts his hips forward. This makes the position very very deep.

Put your hand between your legs and masturbate. Many women find rear-entry positions to be vaginally very stimulating. Supplement the sensations by rubbing your fingers against your clitoris. Your orgasm will be deep and intense.

Royally Screwed

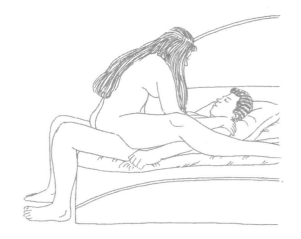

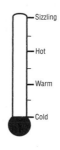

Roll out the red carpet. Tonight you will treat your partner like they're royalty.

The king lies on the bed with his legs hanging over the edge. The queen sits on the royal throne facing him. Her legs are spread out wide in front of her. The king should put his hand around his scepter and guide it deep inside the queen's warm and wonderful castle.

Queens, reach behind you and fondle the royal jewels between your partner's legs. To make the penetration even deeper, lean forward. Run your fingers through his hair. Use your other hand to reach between your legs and manually stimulate your clitoris. Thrust your hips until both you and the king have conquered your greatest heights.

Oh, and use some protection. Unless, of course, you want little princes and princesses running around your kingdom.

Hold Your Fire

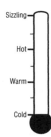

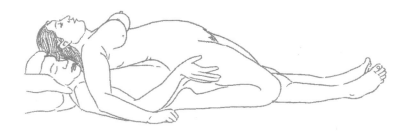

And guys, this position will let you hold your fire really close!

Lie on your back with your legs out straight. Have your partner sit on top, facing your feet, with her legs bent so that her feet are behind her. Slide your woody into her fireplace. Once you have successfully added your fuel to her fire, have your partner lean all the way back until she is resting on your chest.

And now, despite all the warnings you have heard telling you not to do this, it's time to play with fire. Put your hands on your partner's breasts and gently massage them. Rub the palms of your hands against her nipples. Roll the nipple between your thumb and finger. Encourage your partner to put her own irons in her fire and masturbate. Put your arms around your partner and hold your fire while both of you orgasm.

Get Over It!

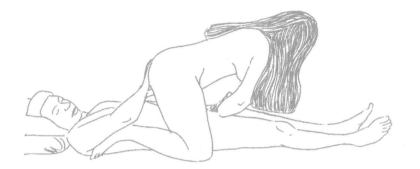
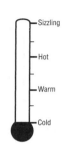

Sizzling

Hot

Warm

Cold

This position, which has each of you manually stimulating your partner, will put both of you over the top. Even though the man is on the bottom.

The man lies comfortably on his back. Ladies, straddle your partner so that your head is hanging over his penis and your bottom is hanging over his head. Loosely wrap your hand around the shaft of your partner's penis and lightly stroke it. Twirl your hand around the head. Briefly wrap your hand around his testicles. And then return to holding the shaft.

Guys, while your partner is stimulating you, you should also be stimulating her. Reach your hand up and stroke between your partner's cheeks. Rub the very sensitive area around her anus. With your other hand, lightly stroke her labia and the areas around her clitoris.

Spend some time simultaneously arousing each other. Decide if you want to take turns reaching your peaks or if you want to climax together. In either case, both of you should intensify the stimulation. Focus on your partner's favorite areas. Use the pressure and pace they love the most. Bring your partner to a satisfying orgasm.

Disappointed that it's all over? Get over it! And, thankfully, you can get over it over and over again!

The Love God

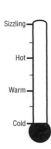

Sizzling

Hot

Warm

Cold

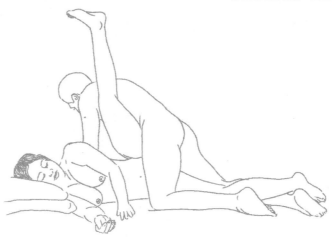

Cupid is the Roman god of love. Eros is the Greek god of love. And your partner is your god of love.

This position looks a little awkward, but it's actually easy to accomplish. The woman lies on her side. The man is kneeling next to her. The woman has one leg between her partner's legs. The other leg is sideways, pointing toward her shoulder.

Guys, check the shaft of your arrow to be sure it's hard and straight. Then shoot your arrow into your partner's target. Thrust your hips forward as you score a direct hit.

Ladies, put your hand down between your legs. Let the heel of your hand rub against your clitoris. At the same time, use two of your fingers to grip the base of your partner's penis. Keep in mind that your partner is likely to find this highly arousing. In fact, it will probably accelerate how quickly he has his orgasm. So keep the grip gentle until you've gotten yourself stimulated and aroused. Then tighten your fingers and enjoy a dual climax.

A Sticky Situation

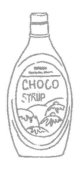

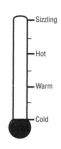

Your partner, your tongue, and some chocolate syrup. A very sticky situation indeed!

Ladies, you and your chocolate syrup will be giving your partner a wonderful fellatio treat. This activity is even better if the chocolate syrup is cold. Start by dripping the syrup on your partner's chest, especially around his nipples. Dart your tongue over the chocolate and lick the skin clean. Put your mouth around each nipple and suck off all the chocolate syrup. Swirl the syrup over your partner's torso from his chest to his groin. Flatten your tongue. Slowly and seductively drag your tongue all around your partner's skin.

Put some drops of chocolate syrup on the head of your partner's penis. Rub the drops around with your fingers and get the head nice and sticky. Ceremoniously lick the chocolate off your fingers before wrapping your mouth around your partner's head. Roll your tongue all over the head of the penis, replacing the stickiness with warm wetness. Drizzle thin lines of the syrup all over the shaft of your partner's penis. With a flat tongue, lick up and down the shaft. Pour on some more chocolate syrup and lower your mouth over the head and as much of the shaft as you can. Rub your tongue all around as you lift and lower your head. If your partner needs additional stimulation, wrap your hand around the shaft and move it up and down simultaneously with your mouth. Continue stroking and licking until your partner has reached chocolate heaven.

Love Seat

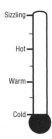

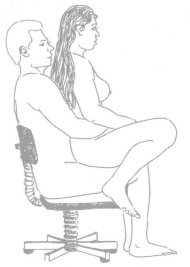

Technically, a love seat is a small couch with enough room to sit two people. Of course, when the woman sits on her partner's lap, even chairs for one can be love seats. We'll prove it with this month's loving chair position.

Guys, sit down comfortably on a chair, couch, or love seat. Have your partner sit in your lap facing the same direction you are facing. Her legs should be bent so that her feet are flat on the cushion next to your legs. Use your hand to guide your penis into your partner's vagina. Put your arms around your partner and pull her to you. Use your hands to lovingly massage your partner's breasts.

Ladies, lean back and rest against your partner's chest. Spread your legs apart as wide as you can. This makes the penetration very deep. It also gives your hand lots of room for masturbation. Use your favorite rubbing technique to arouse and stimulate yourself. Increase the intensity of your masturbation as your partner increases the depth and speed of his thrusts. Try to time your orgasm so that you and your partner can reach your peaks simultaneously.

Wrong-Hand Man

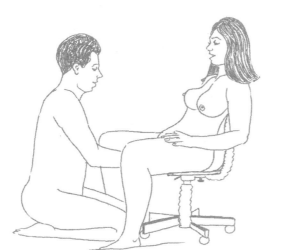

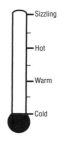

Sizzling

Hot

Warm

Cold

Ladies, your right-hand man is going to be your wrong-hand man for this manual stimulation position. So sit down and relax in your favorite chair.

Guys, spread your partner's legs apart and kneel down between them. Using just your fingertip, lightly write your name on the skin at the top of your partner's inner thigh. Move your fingertips around like you're doodling. The soft, delicate touch is very arousing.

Move your hand over to your partner's vulva. Switch to the hand you don't normally use. If you're right-handed, use your left hand. If you're left-handed, use your right. It might feel a little awkward at first, but stay with it. Sometimes minor changes can have dramatic effects.

Continue stimulating your partner. Tickle the area around her vagina. Stroke your fingers along her labia. Rub your fingers against her clitoris. Prove to your partner that her right-hand man is ambidextrous!

Hot Under the Collar

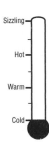

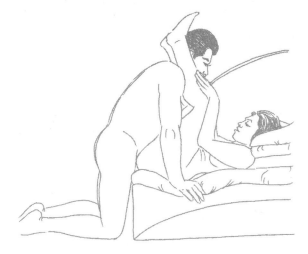

This position will definitely have you hot and bothered. And with your partner's legs around your neck, you'll be hot under the collar too.

Ladies, lie on your back with your legs hanging over the edge of the bed. Lower your hips as far over the edge as you can. This will make it much easier for your partner to penetrate. Have your partner kneel between your legs. Lift your legs in front of him and rest them on his shoulders. Wrap your hand around the shaft of your partner's penis and guide him to your sweet, hot vagina.

Guys, this position allows for very deep penetration. Thrust your hips all the way forward and take full advantage of this. Make eye contact with your partner as you massage her breasts. Encourage her to masturbate. Things will be hot and heavy when both of you reach your peaks!

Birds of a Feather . . .

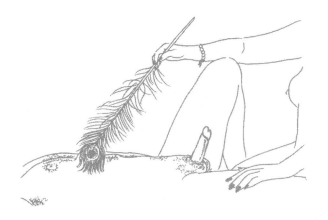

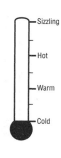

- Sizzling
- Hot
- Warm
- Cold

Birds would be envious of humans if they knew all the things we were doing with their feathers! Ladies, get your feather ready. This activity has you teasing and tantalizing your partner with it until you finally satisfy him with some manual stimulation.

Start by tickling your partner on the neck. Follow this up with some soft kisses. Then, rub the feather against your partner's nipples, arousing them until they're nice and taut. Lower your mouth around the nipple and gently suck on it. Stroke your partner's torso with the feather. Drag it back and forth from one side to the other. The soft touch of the feather is very sensuous.

Rub the feather against the top of your partner's inner thighs. Tickle it against his testicles. Wrap your hand around his testicles and rub the feather up and down the shaft of your partner's penis. Very lightly stroke the feather against the head of your partner's penis. Glide it all around the edge. Tantalize and tease until your partner can't stand it any longer. Then wrap your hand around the shaft and stroke him until he climaxes.

Horsing Around

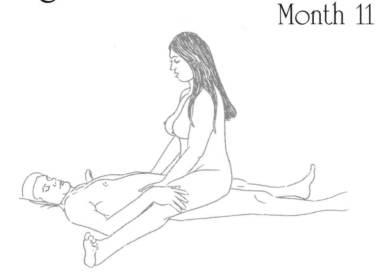

Sizzling

Hot

Warm

Cold

Get ready to mount your partner, ladies, and enjoy a great ride. Have your partner lie on his back with his legs straight out in front of him. Before getting into the saddle, wrap your hand around your partner's penis and stroke it.

Sit down on top of the horse facing your partner. Your legs should be spread apart as wide as you can get them. Start your horse out at a slow trot. Let your hips move back and forth in the saddle matching your horse's gait. Increase the speed to a canter. Rub your hand against your clitoris as your horse starts to gallop. Ride your horse until both of you cross the finish line.

Think you and your horse ride pretty well? You can always consider the equestrian events at the next summer Olympics. Of course, in the meantime, keep practicing!

Man in the Moon

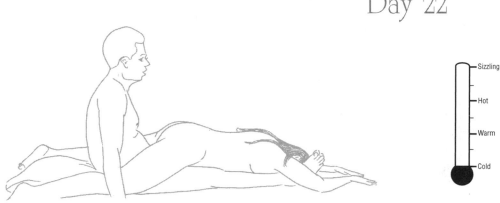

Sizzling

Hot

Warm

Cold

This position will have both of you over the moon with pleasure. So turn off the lights and let the moonlight shine through your windows. A full moon is about to rise.

Ladies, have your partner sit on the bed with his legs out straight in front of him. You'll be lying on your partner, with your head near his feet and your legs out straight behind you. The easiest way to accomplish this position is to start out by sitting on your partner with your legs bent so that your feet are behind you. Use your hand to guide your partner's penis inside of you. Then carefully lean forward until your breasts are rubbing against your partner's legs and your arms are flat on the bed. Remember to take this slow so that you don't hurt your partner. As you lean forward, straighten out your legs behind you. For the deepest penetration, move yourself backward until your vulva is pressed up against your partner's torso.

Guys, when your partner leans forward, watch the full moon rising. Grab her buttocks with your hands and massage them. Lightly stroke the area around her anus. Pull her hips to you as you reach your peak. Then promise her the moon if she'll do this position one more time!

Hot and Tasty

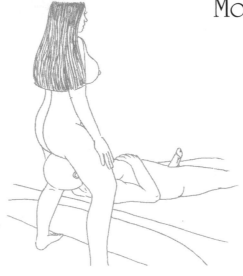

Sizzling

Hot

Warm

Cold

With the help of some magical oil, this cunnilingus position truly can be hot and tasty. Start out at an adult store or Web site and look in the section for sexual oils. Find the flavored oils that get hot when you blow them. Choose the flavor you want and you're ready to get started.

Guys, lie on your back on the bed with your head (the one on your shoulders, this isn't fellatio) at the edge of the bed. Have your partner

stand next to the bed and straddle your face. She should be facing the bed. Put a pillow or two under your head if your partner is tall and you need some additional height.

Using your fingers, rub the oil all over your partner's vulva. Lick the outside of your partner's vagina. The taste of your partner and the oil will combine on your tongue for a tasty treat. Before licking the oil from your partner's

labia, blow on them. Your partner should feel a rush of heat as the oil gets warm. Follow this up by licking the labia, separating them with your tongue as you move up to your partner's clitoris.

Blow and lick the area around your partner's clitoris, applying more oil as desired. Use your hands to hold your partner's hips still while you rub your tongue back and forth. Bring her to a hot and tasty orgasm.

Straddle the Fence

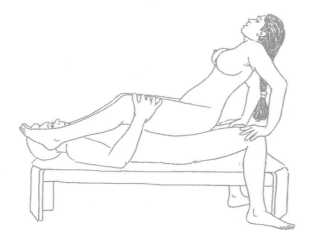

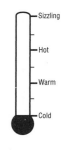

Sizzling

Hot

Warm

Cold

Okay, so maybe a fence isn't quite wide enough to hold you. Instead, find a bench or table that you can straddle.

Guys are on the bottom for this one. Lie on your back with your legs hanging over the sides of the bench. Make sure your feet can touch the floor. It'll make the thrusting easier and stronger.

Ladies, sit on top of your partner facing him. Let your legs straddle the bench while you lower your hips down the shaft of your partner's penis. Lean backward with your arms on the bench behind you. Lift up each leg and place it on your partner's shoulder. Make this tight position even tighter by clenching your vaginal muscles around your partner's penis.

Guys, kiss and nibble your partner's ankles. Feel her smooth silky skin up against your face. Reach forward and use your hand to manually stimulate your partner's clitoris. Because her legs are together, it will be a little challenging to get enough room to move your fingers. So keep the strokes short, but firm. Thrust your hips as you rub your fingers back and forth until both of you have climaxed.

Still on the fence about this position? Try it again and get a second opinion.

Double Cross

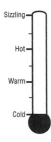

Sizzling

Hot

Warm

Cold

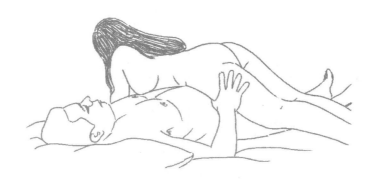

This was originally a sports gambling term that started in the late 1800s. It referred to a player who had promised to throw a game, but in the end, broke his word. So, when you promise your partner that you plan to double-cross him tonight, make sure you keep your promise.

Ladies, have your partner lie on his back with his legs straight in front of him. You'll be lying on top of your partner at a 90 degree angle. This position needs good lubrication, so start by lowering your mouth down over your partner's penis and getting him really wet. Lie down on your tummy sideways on top of your partner. The easiest way to achieve penetration is to turn your hips sideways so that you can line up the entrance of your vagina with the head of your partner's penis. Slide your hips down the shaft and then turn your hips back to where they started and press your legs together behind you.

Like most sideways penetration positions, this one is very tight. Let your partner do most of the thrusting. Rub your hips up against your partner's hips. Slide them around until your clitoris is being stimulated each time your partner thrusts. Grind your hips into your partner as both of you orgasm.

Vibrator Madness

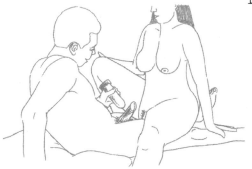

Sizzling

Hot

Warm

Cold

I think the overwhelming sensations created by a vibrator can cause temporary madness in the person being stimulated. Even the strongest minds go crazy from the intense pleasure caused when the sensitive nerve endings are exposed to the millions of tiny jolts. For this intercourse activity, the guys will be inflicting madness on themselves.

Pick a position where the man has access to his testicles and the base of his penis. Rear-entry positions work great. So do positions where the man is sitting with his legs spread apart, the woman is sitting upright, and the woman's legs are not in the way. If you need some help finding a suitable position, use one of the positions listed below.

Guys, no need to wait until intercourse to start using the vibrator. Rub it up against the shaft of your penis. Circle it around the outside edge of the penis head. Let it work its magic on the head's entire surface. Use it on your partner to increase her stimulation too. Sometimes this can be almost as arousing as using it on yourself.

Once intercourse has started and you've established penetration, hold the vibrator against your testicles. If possible, depending on her position, rub the vibrator against your partner's labia and clitoris. The indirect vibrations that you'll feel on your penis are still very stimulating. As your arousal increases and you start to approach your climax, move the vibrator to the base of your penis. The direct stimulation you feel each time you thrust will take you over the brink to a quick, but happy, ending.

Suggested positions: Month 1/Day 20 — Snake in the Grass; Month 3/Day 14 — Who Let the Dog Out?; Month 5/Day 16 — Sit Tight; Month 6/Day 19 — Couch Potato; Month 11/Day 11 — What's Cooking.

Face Value

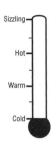

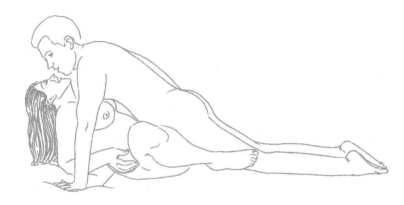

Our faces tell so much about us. We use them, sometimes inadvertently, to express our emotions. We use them to show friendship and warmth. We use them as a reflection of ourselves. The face has an extraordinary value that gives face-to-face positions a wonderful intimacy.

For this position, the woman is on her back with her arms bent behind her and her weight on her elbows. Her legs should be bent so that her feet are on their sides. The man lies between the woman's open legs. His weight rests on his arms in front of him. His legs are straight behind him.

Because the woman's shoulders and head are elevated, this position offers great face-to-face opportunities. Make eye contact with your partner and smile at them. Truly look into their eyes and emotionally connect with them. Lovingly kiss your partner. If you can hold your weight on one arm, fondly caress your partner's face. Whisper to each other. Tell your partner how wonderful they are and how blessed you are to be with them.

Thrust your hips until you orgasm. Continue to hold each other and cuddle even after intercourse is over.

Gone Fishing

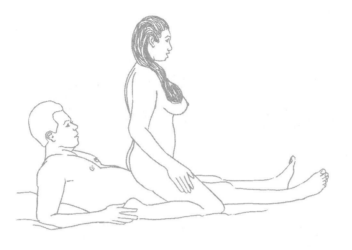

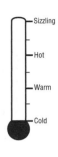

Sizzling

Hot

Warm

Cold

Bait your hook, ladies. You've got a big fish to catch! Start with your partner dressed so you can do some fly fishing. Rub your hand up against his pants until your partner is hard. Then unzip his fly so he can take them off.

Have your partner lie on his back. His arms should be bent behind him with his weight resting on his elbows. Straddle your partner facing his feet. Your legs should be bent so that your feet are behind you. Lure your partner by rubbing the head of his penis against your vulva — you need to be very wet. You've cast your line. Now lower your hips and reel him in. Enjoy the tightness of this position. You've got a big fish in your little pond.

Place your hand between your legs. Tickle your partner's testicles with your fingers. Fondle and caress them. Rub your hand across your clitoris. Use a circular motion to get yourself aroused. Switch to rubbing back and forth when you and your partner are ready to orgasm.

And while there may be many fish in the sea, let your partner know that you're very happy with the fish you've caught!

Holding the Torch

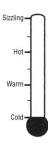

Sizzling

Hot

Warm

Cold

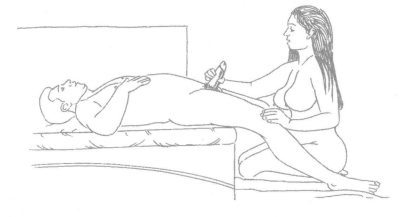

Ladies, set your partner's torch on fire with this manual stimulation position. Your partner needs to lie down on the bed with his legs hanging over the edge. Spread his knees apart and kneel down on the floor between them.

Start by blowing on the flames. Lick all around the head and shaft of your partner's penis. A little water won't put out this fire. It'll just help make the torch slippery.

Put one hand on the base of the torch. Use the other hand to rub all around the head. Move your hand up and down the shaft. Do a few slow strokes followed by a few quick strokes. Then stop stroking and just rub the head. Continue alternating between slow strokes, fast strokes, and rubbing the head. The variety of sensations will drive your partner crazy! Let him feel the burn!

As your partner's arousal increases, firmly move your hand up and down the shaft and head of the penis at a steady pace. Continue stimulating him until the torch has been extinguished.

It Takes Two

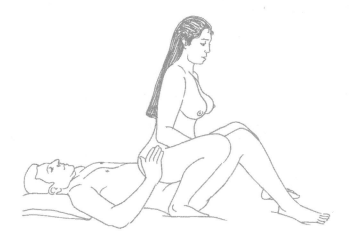

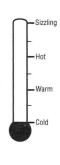

There are no two ways about it. Two can play this game. So let me tell you a thing or two about this position.

The man lies on his back with his legs bent at the knees. The woman sits on top of him facing his feet with her legs bent so that her feet are flat on the bed next to her partner's hips.

With your legs bent, guys, this position is great for strong powerful thrusts. At the same time, use your hands to caress your partner's lower back and sides.

Ladies, reach down between your legs and wrap your hands around your partner's testicles. Roll them around between your fingers. Use your other hand to stimulate your clitoris. As you approach your peak, move your fingers from your partner's testicles to the base of his penis and give it a soft squeeze. Your chances of peaking together have just increased two hundred percent!

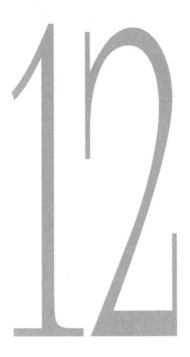

MONTH 12

Day 1. Old Dogs, New Tricks

Day 2. Cathisophobes Need

Not Apply

Day 3. Man's Best Friend?

Day 4. Kiss Off

Day 5. Cause and Effect

Day 6. Happy Hour

Day 7. Pulsating Tongue

Day 8. Day at the Beach

Day 9. Half-Cocked

Day 10. Jungle Love

Day 11. Lap Dance

Day 12. Love Is Blind

Day 13. Sacked!

Day 14. Greased Lightning

Day 15. Bring to Your Knees

Day 16. Say "Cheese"

Day 17. Opposites Attract

Day 18. Self-Service Lane

Day 19. Dog Days

Day 20. Light My Fire

Day 21. Headlock

Day 22. Dance with the Devil

Day 23. Playing Cat and Mouse

Day 24. Sidewinder

Day 25. The Language of Love

Day 26. In Your Wildest Dreams

Day 27. Come to a Head

Day 28. My Lips Are Sealed

Day 29. Hard Up

Day 30. Going Out with a Bang

Old Dogs, New Tricks

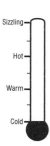

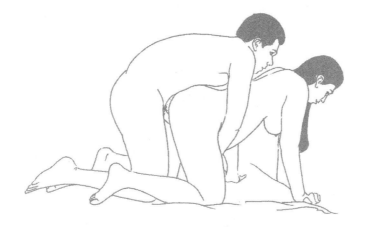

Guys, this is your chance to prove to your partner that old dogs really can learn new tricks! And what better way to do this than with a good manual stimulation position.

Guys, have your partner get on her hands and knees, doggy-style. You will also be on your hands and knees behind her. Start by reaching around your partner and putting your hands on her breasts. Let your legs hold your weight. It's a lot more comfortable for the woman if she doesn't have you resting your upper body weight against her. Because of the position of your partner, you can feel the fullness of her breasts. Massage and knead them with your hands. Lean forward and kiss her on the back and shoulders.

Leaving your arm wrapped around your partner, take one hand and bring it down to her vulva. Take the other hand and put it between her legs from behind her. Use the front hand to stroke her labia and clitoris. Use the back hand to insert a finger, or two if your partner likes it, into her vagina. Don't thrust your finger in and out. Instead, apply pressure to the sides of the vagina, particularly the front. Simultaneously rub the clitoris back and forth with the other hand. Your partner will experience a deep and powerful orgasm from the dual stimulation.

Cathisophobes Need Not Apply

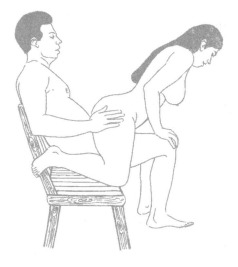

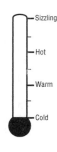

Sizzling

Hot

Warm

Cold

If you're afraid of sitting (cathisophobic), then this chair position is not for you. Of course, you also won't be interested if you're coitophobic (afraid of intercourse), aphenphosmphobic (afraid to be touched), medorthophobic (afraid of erect penises), or heterophobic (afraid of the opposite sex). But have no fear. This is a fun and enjoyable position for everybody else.

For this position, the man sits comfortably in a chair or on a couch. Ladies, start by some soft kisses to your partner's lips. Then sit on your partner's lap facing the same direction. Your legs should be bent so that your feet are behind you. Hope you're not hygrophobic (afraid of wetness and moisture) because good sex requires good slippery lubrication. Once your partner has penetrated, place your

hands on your partner's knees and lean forward.

Thrust your hips up and down your partner's shaft. Thermophobics (afraid of heat) are going to start getting nervous because things are getting very hot. So unless you're hedonophobic (afraid of pleasure), continue thrusting until both of you orgasm.

Man's Best Friend?

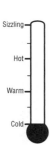

Sizzling

Hot

Warm

Cold

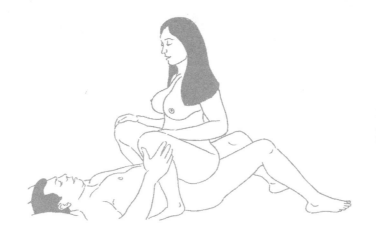

Why is the dog a man's best friend when every day he gets so much pleasure from his partner's soft, furry pussycat? The pussycat has some wonderful and endearing qualities that can't be matched by any breed of dog. So, ladies, use this position to demonstrate to your partner just how great your pussycat can behave.

Have your partner lie on his back with his legs bent at the knees. Facing your partner, straddle him and rub his penis against your furry pubic hair. Do you feel him arching his back and trying to thrust his hips? He is being converted to a pussycat lover already.

Lift your hips so that your partner's penis is rubbing against the opening of your vagina. Using your hand to hold the shaft still, lower your hips so that just the head has penetrated.

Ask your partner if he's still a dog lover. If he says yes, pull the head back out and resume foreplay. If he says no, move your hand and let his penis slide all the way inside of you.

Take your partner's hand and guide it between your legs. Keep your fingers on top of his as you show him where and how you want to be stimulated. Let out a big meow as both of you reach your peaks.

Kiss Off

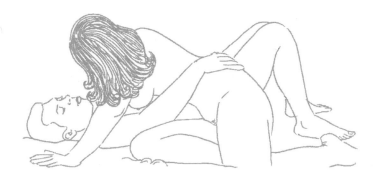

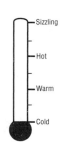

Ladies, this is a great fellatio activity that will have you kissing your partner from his head down to his head. You'll notice this doesn't include having to kiss his ass.

This activity works best if your partner is lying on his back. Start by kissing him on the face, and not just on the lips. Kiss him very gently on his eyelids. Some men will be surprised to find that the delicate touch is arousing. Turn up the heat by indulging in some mouth-to-mouth passionate kissing.

Use your tongue and tickle your partner at the base of his neck. Drag your tongue to his ear and nibble on his earlobe. Give him lots of small kisses down his neck and chest. Then, seal your mouth around his nipple and gently suck on it, rubbing it back and forth with your tongue. While stimulating one nipple with your mouth, use your hand to stimulate the other one.

Use small kisses again to get from your partner's chest down to his groin. Lightly drag your fingernails against his skin while you're kissing him. Seductively, but chastely, kiss the very tip of his penis. It promises so much, but delivers so little! Tease your partner a little bit longer. Open your lips slightly and let less than an inch of his head inside your mouth. Close your lips and run your tongue around it. Follow this by finally taking the entire head inside your mouth. You're hot and wet. Waiting for this drove him crazy, but it feels so good!

Wrap your hand around your partner's shaft. Simultaneously lift and lower your mouth and hand up and down the shaft of his penis until you're ready to kiss this one goodbye.

Cause and Effect

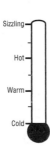

Sizzling
Hot
Warm
Cold

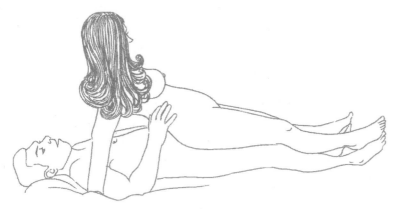

Ladies, you will primarily be the cause. Your partner will primarily feel the effect.

Cause: Approach your partner while he's watching TV. While you unzip his pants, tell him that you're very hot for him.
Effect: Your partner gets a hard-on.

Cause: Take off your clothes and leave a trail of clothes to your bedroom.
Effect: Your partner will follow you.

Cause: Have your partner lie down on the bed with his legs straight in front of him. Sit down on top of your partner, facing his feet.
Effect: Your partner feels a rush of heat as he finds his penis encircled by your warm, wet vagina.

Cause: Clench your legs together and rest them on top of your partner's legs.
Effect: Lots and lots of skin contact and a very tight penetration.

Cause: Lean backward toward your partner with your arms behind you.
Effect: The penetration just got significantly deeper.

Cause: You thrust your hips up and down your partner's shaft causing friction while simultaneously rubbing one hand against your clitoris.
Effect: Wonderfully satisfying orgasms.

Happy Hour

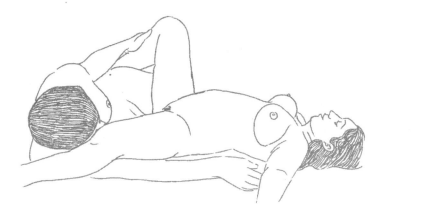

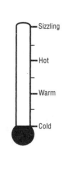

Guys, time to make your partner a happy camper. Tonight, take your time and convince your partner that this is the best happy hour she has ever attended.

Lie down on your side. In order for your partner to have enough room, you'll need your back to be near the edge of the bed. Your partner is on her back, perpendicular to you. One of her legs should be over your hips. Her other leg should be spread wide open to her side. Use your hand to guide your penis inside of her as she moves her hips toward you.

Use your hand to manually stimulate your partner. With her legs spread so wide apart, you have lots of room to maneuver your fingers. Try to coordinate your thrusting and stroking so that you hit her most sensitive areas while you are deep inside of her. Increase the pressure and pace until both of you experience many happy returns.

Pulsating Tongue

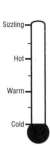

Sizzling

Hot

Warm

Cold

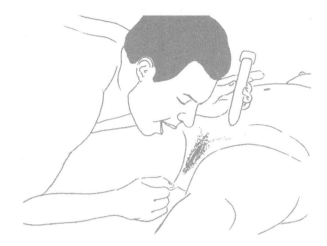

This can only describe one activity. And that is when the man performs cunnilingus on his partner while simultaneously using the vibrator. It's a powerful combination that can produce multiple, deep orgasms for many women!

Start by using the vibrator on your partner's breasts. Make a circle around the largest part of your partner's breast. Move the vibrator toward the center, making the circle smaller and smaller, until you're rubbing the vibrator against your partner's nipple. Move the vibrator down to her tummy and lower your mouth over the nipple. Your soft, wet, hot mouth after the pulsating vibrator is very arousing!

Drag the vibrator against your partner's stomach and lower torso, while steadily moving toward her genitals. Rub the vibrator all around your partner's pubic hair. Then move it over the labia and to her vagina. Insert just the tip into your partner's vagina and roll it around the outer edge. At the same time, lower your mouth around her clitoral area. Rub your tongue back and forth over her clitoris. The combination of the vibrator and your tongue will quickly cause your partner to orgasm. So, don't quit until she's had a few!

A Day at the Beach

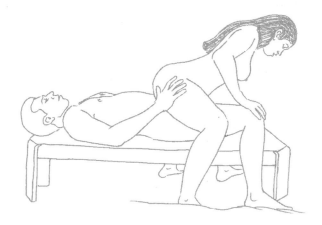

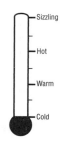

Sizzling

Hot

Warm

Cold

The sun, the sand, and the water. There's nothing like a day at the beach! So grab your partner, a towel, and a reclining beach chair. Get ready for some sun and fun.

Guys, you're the lifeguard. Let your partner know she doesn't seem to be breathing. A little mouth-to-mouth resuscitation is definitely needed. Pull her close to you and kiss her very softly and sweetly on her lips.

Then lie down on the beach chair so that your legs straddle both sides.

Ladies, you can't bury your partner's head in the sand, but you can bury him in your mouth. Lower your mouth down his head and shaft. Swish your tongue back and forth like waves on the beach.

Apply some suntan oil to your partner's penis. You would hate for his very sensitive skin to get burned!

Sit down on top of your partner, facing away from him. Let your hand guide his penis into your beach bag. Your legs should also be straddling the sides of the beach chair. Make the position tight by leaning all the way forward. Reach your hand between your partner's legs and play with his beach balls. Ride the waves until both of you have reached high tide.

Half-Cocked

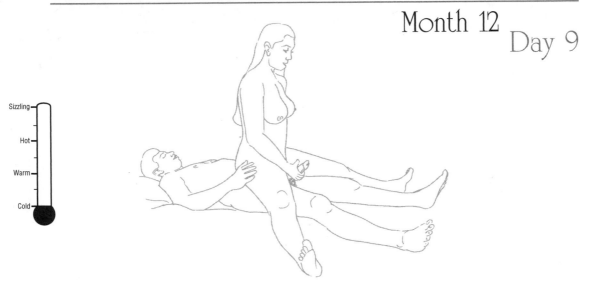

Sizzling —

Hot —

Warm —

Cold —

When a gun is half-cocked, it means the hammer is raised halfway and locked into position so that the trigger cannot be pulled. Ladies, if your partner is half-cocked, use this position to get him fully erect and pleasantly pull his trigger.

Ladies, you can feel cocky about this manual stimulation position. Your partner lies on his back. You sit on your partner's torso facing his feet with his penis upright between your thighs. Squeeze your thighs together so that your partner's penis is surrounded by your soft skin. Flex and relax your thigh muscles to alternate between a strong and weak squeeze.

Open your legs and move back a little bit so that your hands have room to move around. Start with one hand at the base of your partner's penis and slide it up the shaft and off the head. As soon as your hand has left the end of the penis, repeat this same motion with your other hand. Continue alternating between hands.

Periodically, take a short break. Wrap one hand around your partner's testicles while the other hand moves up and down the shaft of the penis. Then, resume alternating both hands up the shaft and off the head. When your partner is close to reaching his peak, he might want you to switch to using just one hand until he orgasms. And that's okay. After all, worse than going off half-cocked is not going off at all.

Jungle Love

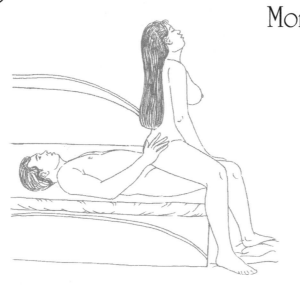

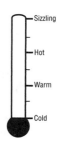

Sizzling

Hot

Warm

Cold

You'll have to take off your loincloths for this hot and steamy jungle position. Jungle fever has never felt so good!

The law of the jungle dictates that the man lies down on the bed. His legs should be together and hanging over the edge. The woman sits on top, facing the man's feet. Her legs should be spread open and bent to the floor. The jungle is a very wet, tropical area. Lubrication shouldn't be a problem.

Guys, you'll be doing the lion's share of the thrusting for this one. Push your feet against the floor for leverage. Reach forward with your hands and stroke your lover's hips and lower back. Encourage her to masturbate. Continue thrusting until you and your partner feel like the king and queen of the jungle.

Lap Dance

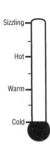

Sizzling
Hot
Warm
Cold

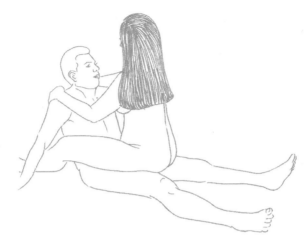

Ladies, turn on the music and get ready to turn your room into a strip club for one. If you've ever wondered what it's like to parade around while seductively taking off your clothes, you're about to find out. Of course, you're only doing this for an audience of one — your partner. So if you're a little self-conscious, just remember that men love strip routines and lap dances. And he'll love yours!

Slowly and seductively dance for your partner while taking off items of clothing. Start with the items that reveal the least. Leave the panties for last. Each time you take off an article of clothing, dance around for your partner. After you've taken off your bra, rub your hands all over your breasts. Let your fingers stroke your nipples. Your partner will want to stroke himself.

When you've removed everything, use dance movements that tantalize and tease. Slowly lift and lower your legs so that your partner can catch glimpses of your soft, wet vulva. Turn your back to him and bend over to give him a great view of your bottom.

If he hasn't already done so, help your partner remove his clothes. Have him sit on the bed or floor with his legs spread open in front of him. Facing him, lower yourself all the way down onto your partner's lap so that he can be in as deep as possible. Squeeze your legs together around your partner's hips to make things tight. Let your hips dance around while you thrust up and down his shaft. Hold your partner close as each of you reach your peaks.

Love Is Blind

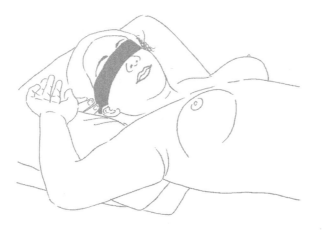

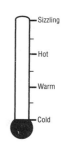

Sizzling

Hot

Warm

Cold

Or in this case, guys, your lover is blindfolded. Cover her eyes and have her lie down on the bed. Women can be kind of sneaky sometimes, so make sure her blindfold is tight enough that she can't peek. Look around your room and gather up a variety of textures that you can rub against your partner. Try to find things that contain leather, silk, fur, velvet, and anything else that feels interesting. Rub each piece of fabric, one at a time, against your partner. Let her feel it against her arms, breasts, and legs. See if she can guess the type of fabric it is without touching it with her hands.

Use the different fabrics and randomly rub them against your partner's body. Use the silk on one of her arms. Then rub the leather on one of her legs. Follow this with the fur against the other leg. Keep your partner guessing which fabric you'll use and which part of her body you will be touching. Periodically, drag the fabric across her vulva as you move from one spot on her body to another. It's a tease, and it will heighten her anticipation.

Rub each fabric against your partner's vulva. Once she has tried them all, let her choose which fabric she would like you to use while you manually stimulate her. Of course, if none of them are very arousing for her, she can also elect for you to use your bare hand. Rub the fabric against your partner's clitoris. You might need to apply more pressure with your fingers than usual. Your partner will let you know. Continue working the fabric back and forth until your partner climaxes.

Sacked!

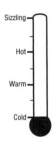

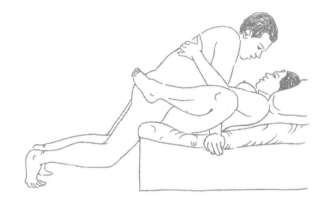

No, guys, you haven't been fired! And although you'll be hitting the sack, you certainly won't be sleeping.

Have your partner sack out on the bed. She should be on her back with her legs hanging over the edge. Stand between your partner's legs. Extend your legs behind you while you lean forward with your arms on the bed. Line yourself up and rub the head of your penis all around on your partner's vulva. Make sure everything is good and wet.

Insert just the tip of your penis into your partner's vagina. Start with a few shallow thrusts. She wants to feel you deep inside of her and will lift her hips to help make this happen. Tease her for a bit. Then slowly lean forward and slide all the way inside.

Ladies, bend your legs so that your feet are flat against your partner's hips. This gives your partner more room to lean forward and allows for the deepest penetration. Slide your hand between your partner and your clitoris so you can masturbate. Since you won't have a lot of room, let your partner's hips bump against your hand each time he thrusts. He'll find it erotic and you'll find the extra pressure will help you orgasm.

Greased Lightning

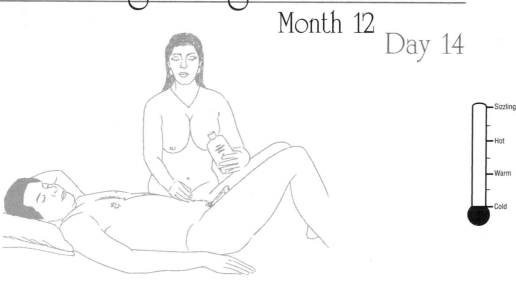

Sizzling

Hot

Warm

Cold

Ladies, get out some oil or lotion for this manual stimulation activity. Sex oils can be found in many different scents, colors, and consistencies. Select a product that has an aroma you think your partner will like and that you think will complement the ambience. Some scents are designed to be relaxing while others are formulated to energize. So pick a mood and a product and get started.

Generously coat your hands with the oil and massage the skin around the base of your partner's penis. (Don't actually touch his penis yet.) Pour some oil into the palm of your hand and wrap it around your partner's testicles. Feel them slide back and forth in your hand as they get slippery. Pour some oil onto the head of your partner's penis. This feels especially nice if the oil has been warmed up ahead of time. Use the palm of your hand to rub the oil all around the head. Notice how soft the skin feels against your fingers as you use them to stroke the head.

Apply oil to the shaft of the penis. Wrap your hand around it and stroke from the base to the head. Your hand should glide very smoothly over the slick skin. You're probably producing less friction because of the oil, so you might want to tighten your grip just a bit. Ask your partner to let you know what feels right. Continue stroking from base to head, using two hands if you want, until your partner climaxes.

Bring to Your Knees

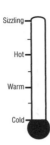

Sizzling

Hot

Warm

Cold

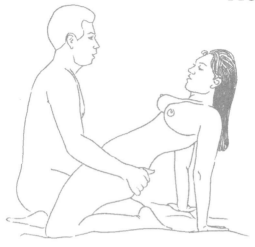

In 1936, Dolores Ibarruri, a Spanish politician, made a speech during a radio broadcast during the Spanish Civil War. She was the first person to make the claim that it's better to die on your feet than to live on your knees. I'm not convinced that the men who kneel down for this position are going to agree with her.

So, ladies, bring your partner to his knees. And just to prove this isn't about subservience, facing your partner, kneel down in front of him. Wrap your arms around him and give him a warm, wet kiss on his lips. He'll willingly be submissive for anything else you have in mind.

Sit down on your partner's lap with your legs bent so that your feet are behind you. Use your hand to guide your partner's penis into your vagina. Scoot your bottom all the way forward so that your vulva is pressed up against him. This will allow you to take every last bit of your partner deep inside of you. Put your arms behind you and slowly lean backward. Clench your vaginal muscles to make this position even tighter.

Guys, use your hands to caress, tickle, and stroke your partner's breasts. Rub the nipple back and forth between your thumb and finger. Pull her hips to you as you climax.

Say "Cheese"

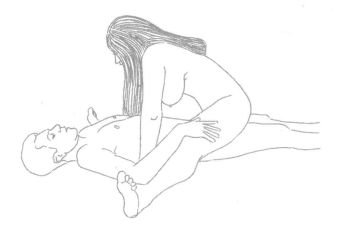

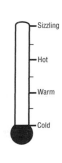

Sizzling

Hot

Warm

Cold

One-hour processing might not be enough for this position. Once you and your partner get in that darkroom, you never know what might develop!

For this position, the man lies on his back with his legs straight in front of him. Ladies, sit down on top of your partner, facing him. Spread your legs apart as wide as you can. Lean forward toward your partner. Enjoy the sensations as you feel your partner deep inside of you.

Focus on your partner. No negatives on this film. Just warm, loving thoughts and actions. Run your fingers through his hair. Stroke his cheeks. Caress his mouth and chin. If you can, lean forward far enough to lightly kiss your partner. Start by simply brushing your lips against his and steadily increase the intensity. Grind your hips into your partner while you thrust until both of you have run out of film.

For the adventurous: Use your digital camera to get some X-rated pictures. Take turns erotically posing and snapping pictures of each other. You can delete any pictures you take from the camera once you're finished, so let loose. Try different angles to get some interesting pictures during intercourse. Getting in front of the camera, even if nobody will ever see the pictures, can be highly arousing and stimulating for many couples.

Opposites Attract

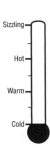

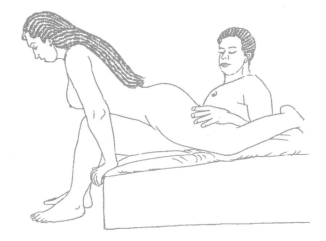

Regardless of how many things you can't agree on, your love of great sex will always give you something in common. So enjoy this position of opposites knowing that you're not always that different from each other.

For some couples, this position is new. For others, it's old. Some will do it in bright light; others prefer sex in the dark. Some couples like sex to be loud; others like it quiet. But there are a few things most couples can agree on. Wet is definitely better than dry. And hot is much better than cold!

For this position, the man is on the bottom and the woman is on the top. The man is face up and the woman is face down. The woman's head is by the man's feet and the man's head is by the woman's feet. The man likes his partner soft; the woman likes her partner hard.

So, ladies, climb on so you can get off. Thrust your hips forward and backward so your partner can slide in and out. Vary your thrusts between deep and shallow, fast and slow, strong and weak. Both of you should feel good as you reach your sexual highs.

Self-Service Lane

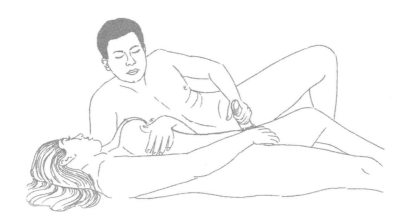

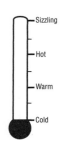

Although this position has you servicing yourself, there's no reason why you can't give yourself the full-service treatment.

Lie down next to each other. The man should be on his side so that he's facing his partner. The woman should be on her back so that she'll have enough room to spread her legs open.

Just because you're not sexually satisfying each other doesn't mean that you can't please each other. Make sure you have lots of eye contact and skin contact as you masturbate. Talk to each other. Take turns so that one of you masturbates while the other one watches.

Guys, suck on your partner's breasts while she is stimulating herself. Rub your tongue around the nipple. Gently bite it.

When it's your turn to masturbate, have your partner do the same for you. Rub the head of your penis up against her skin while you stroke the shaft.

Intimacy does not have to mean intercourse. Since satisfying your partner is not your primary concern, this position is great for paying attention to the small details that help make sex wonderful.

Dog Days

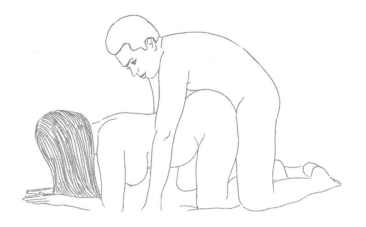

Sizzling

Hot

Warm

Cold

These are the hottest days of July and August named after Sirius, the dog star. During ancient times, the overbearing heat was thought to have been caused by the heliacal rising of Sirius. The Romans called this time *dies caniculares*, which was later translated as dog days.

But no matter what month it is and which stars are rising and falling, make this a dog day with this hot rear-entry position.

This is a fairly standard doggy-style position. The man is on his hands and knees. The woman is in front of the man and also starts on her hands and knees. She then bends her arms and leans forward so that her weight is on her elbows. To make the position particularly tight, the woman should put her legs together. This will put the man's legs on the outside.

Guys, put your hand down at the base of your penis. As you thrust your hips forward and back, wrap your fingers around the shaft of your penis. The firm grip of your fingers stroking your penis plus the feel of your partner's vulva against your hand will intensify the sensations and accelerate your orgasm. Try to pace yourself so that your partner has time to stimulate herself to orgasm too.

Light My Fire

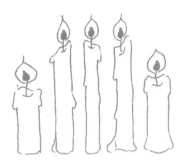

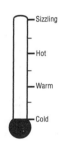

This is a very romantic intercourse activity. Many of you have probably done it before. Light a candle and have sex by candlelight. Have you ever noticed how candles completely alter the ambience of a room? A candlelight dinner for two is much more intimate than just a dinner for two. When the lights go off and the candles are lit, our moods and attitudes improve. Even if sometimes it's only temporarily.

Start out with lots of cuddling and foreplay. Lie next to each other, kissing and caressing. Talk about wonderful times you've spent together in the past and times you want to share with your partner in the future. Remind yourselves how nice it is to truly pull away from your busy schedule and connect heart to heart with your partner. It's a painless and enjoyable activity that many couples don't engage in frequently enough.

Choose a position for intercourse that includes lots of skin contact and eye contact. Positions where the woman is lying on top of her partner are good. So are variations of the missionary position. If you need some help finding a great position, try one of the suggestions listed below. Each of you should be certain that your partner experiences full satisfaction and pleasure.

Romance your partner before, during, and after intercourse. Once the candles have been blown out, you can resume your regular life.

Suggested positions: Month 1/Day17 — Seeing Stars; Month 3/Day 1 — To Have and to Hold; Month 5/Day 10 — Laid to Rest; Month 8/Day 24 — So into You; Month 9/Day 13 — Heart to Heart.

Headlock

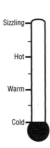

Sizzling
Hot
Warm
Cold

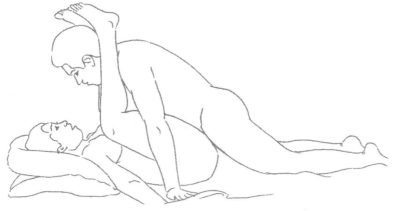

In traditional wrestling, a headlock occurs when you have your arm around your opponent's neck. But in this sexual variation of the sport, you lock your opponent's neck with your feet.

Guys, you need to pin your partner to the mat for this position. With your partner on her back, assume a missionary pose between her legs. Lift her legs in front of your chest as you lean forward and slide your penis inside of her. The further you can lean forward, the deeper the penetration will be. Of course, this also depends on how limber your partner is and how close to her chest she can comfortably get her legs.

Ladies, gently squeeze your partner's head between your legs. Squeeze your vaginal muscles together to give that head a headlock too. Keep your partner locked up until both of you have reached your peaks.

Dance with the Devil

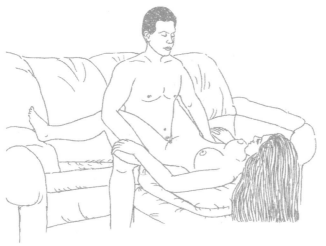

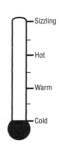

You don't need an excuse to dance with the devil tonight. Just do it for the hell of it.

For this position, the devil sits on a bench with his legs straddling both sides. Make sure his feet can reach the floor. The woman lies down on the bench with her legs over her partner's hips. A pillow or two under her bottom can be used for additional support if desired. Guys, use your hand to hold your penis steady while your partner moves her hips toward you. Watch as it enters her vagina and slides inside of her.

Put your hands on your partner's hips and pull her to you. For the deepest penetration, her vulva should be as close to you as she can get it. Although your partner can move her hips, you should do most of the thrusting. Push your feet off the floor and rock your hips forward and backward. Use your hand to manually stimulate your partner at the same time.

Continue dancing until all hell breaks loose and you've paid the devil his due.

Playing Cat and Mouse

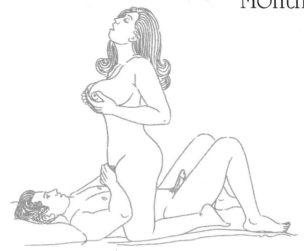

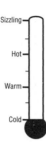

Sizzling

Hot

Warm

Cold

Guys, your partner has the pussy, but you get to play the cat for this manual stimulation position. So, lie on your back. Have your partner straddle you with her chest over your head and her feet by your legs. Make sure your hand can comfortably reach between your partner's legs. If possible, position your partner so that you can reach her breasts with your mouth.

Play cat and mouse with your partner. Very lightly rub your fingers on your partner's vulva. Gradually increase the pressure until you feel your partner's arousal increasing. Then stop moving your hand. Kiss and lick your partner's breasts. Run a finger down her cleavage. Resume stimulating your partner's vulva with your hand.

Again, move your fingers around, steadily increasing the intensity. When you feel her responses start to strengthen, pull your hand back and lower the level of stimulation.

Continue playing cat and mouse until your partner can't stand it any longer. Then continue stimulating her until you bring her to a powerful orgasm.

Sidewinder

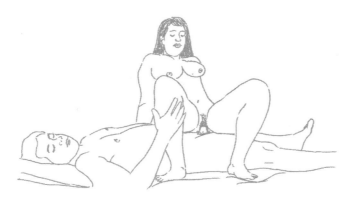

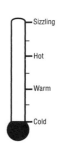

Sizzling

Hot

Warm

Cold

Ladies, you are the snake charmer for this position. Have your partner lie on his back with his legs straight in front of him. Hum some snake charmer music while you move your hands around and get your partner's snake to rise.

Lower your mouth over your partner's penis and get the head and shaft wet.

This is a water snake, so we want to make sure both of you have plenty of liquids available.

Sit down sideways on top of your partner. Your legs should be bent so that your feet are flat on the bed next to your partner's hip. Use your hand to guide the snake to your warm, wet snake hole. Put your arms

behind you and lean backward. Constrict your vaginal muscles around your partner's penis as you thrust your hips. Spread your knees apart so that you can put one of your hands between your legs and masturbate. Continue thrusting until the snake has released its venom.

The Language of Love

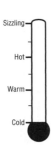

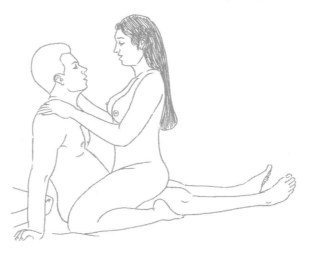

Love. Amour. Amor. Amore. Liebe.

It doesn't matter where you live or what language you speak. The language of love transcends all borders and barriers. For this loving position, use no words to communicate with your partner. Express your feelings and emotions through intimacy and sweet gestures.

Guys, you'll be sitting on the bed or floor with your legs straight in front of you. Your partner will be sitting on your lap facing you. Her legs should be bent so that her feet are behind her. Use your hands to help guide your partner's hips over the head of your penis and down the shaft.

Put your hand behind your partner's head and pull her face to yours for a kiss. Kiss her lips, cheeks, nose, and eyelids. Put your hands behind her back. Use long delicate strokes to caress her skin while you pull her breasts against your chest. Put your hands on your partner's hips to help lift and lower her while she thrusts.

Just because you're not speaking doesn't mean the room needs to be quiet. Moans and sighs are encouraged. And feel free to let out a scream as you orgasm.

In Your Wildest Dreams

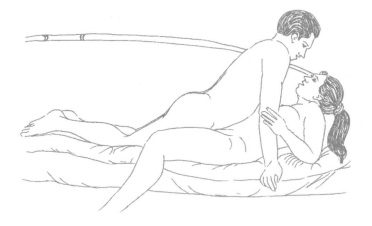

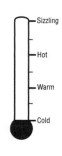

We're talking about your wildest daydreams! A few months ago the guys had to divulge their secret fantasies. Now, ladies, it's time for you to take your turn.

For this position, the woman is on her back with her arms bent behind her so that her weight is on her elbows. This will elevate her head and shoulders and make it much easier to whisper to her partner about her deepest desires. The woman needs to be near the edge of the bed so that one leg can hang over the side. Her other leg is bent so that her foot is flat on the bed close to her bottom.

The man is on his knees between the woman's legs. When he leans forward onto his arms, he'll be able to kiss his partner. Because of the woman's bent leg, this position is very deep. The leg hanging over the bed changes the angle by pulling down on some of the muscles. The net result is a tight, deep penetration. The man should thrust his hips all the way forward to fully enjoy all the benefits.

Ladies, tell your partner some of your fantasies. It might feel a bit uncomfortable and awkward when you first start, but keep going. Your partner loves to hear your private sexual thoughts. And depending on how outlandish or tame these fantasies are, he might be able to make some of your wild dreams come true!

Come to a Head

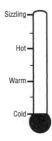

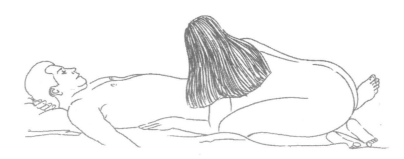

Ladies, unless your partner is a little touched in the head, this fellatio position will make his head spin!

Have your partner lie on his back on the bed. Sit or kneel next to your partner by his hips. Lean over and make sure he's not hanging his head. This position doesn't work if we don't get a heads-up.

Time to use your head. Lower your mouth down around your partner's penis. Lift and lower it a few times to get the head and shaft wet and slippery. Stick out your tongue and drag it up and down the shaft. Each time you get to the top, circle all around the edge of the head. Sometimes after you've licked around the edge, lower your mouth over the whole head and shaft. After just using your tongue, it feels warm and wet when you use your whole mouth again. Then go back to using just the tongue. It's a tease and it works! It builds up his anticipation and heightens his sensations. Eventually, wrap your hand around the shaft and your mouth around the head. Stroke the shaft with your hand while you lift and lower your mouth. You'll know when this has all gone to his head.

My Lips Are Sealed

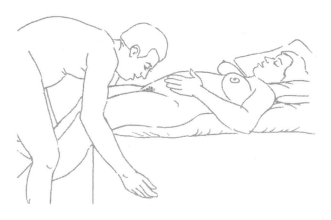

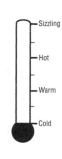

For this cunnilingus position, the woman lies on her back with her legs hanging over the edge of the bed. Guys, spread your partner's legs apart and stand between them. Lick your lips. Then bend down with your mouth between your partner's legs and lick her lips.

While your tongue is busy reading your partner's lips, use your finger to stimulate other areas. Get your finger wet by inserting it into your partner's vagina. Rub it around the edge of the vagina and on the area around the vagina. Make sure it stays wet so it can slide smoothly against your partner's skin.

Spread your partner's lips apart with your tongue. Rub your tongue up and down the area between her labia. Seal your lips around the clitoral area. Rub your partner's clitoris with your tongue. Try a variety of techniques to see which one works best from this angle. Move your tongue in circles, back and forth, and up and down. You'll know which ones are working best by your partner's reaction. Use her favorite techniques on her hot spots until she climaxes.

Hard Up

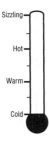

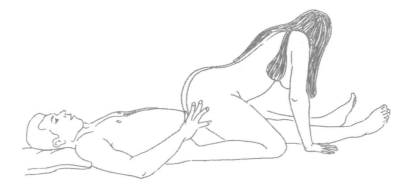

Guys, this is no time for playing hard to get. We all know a hard man is good to find and you're no exception. So there's only one thing that should be getting hard. And I don't think you'll be hard pressed to figure out what it is.

Ladies, hopefully your partner is not too hardheaded and will willingly lie down on his back with his legs straight in front of him. Straddle your partner facing his feet with your legs bent so that your feet are behind you. Wrap your hand around his hard-on and guide it inside your vagina. Spread your legs apart so that your vulva is bumping up against his rocks and his hard place. Lean forward, toward his feet, as far as you can.

Reach your hand between your partner's legs and play a little hardball. Fondle his testicles. Roll them around between your fingers. I don't think there will be any hard feelings if you use your hand to masturbate.

In this position, thrust your hips backward and forward rather than up and down. It'll be much more pleasurable for both of you. Continue thrusting until your partner has produced a hard copy of his work. This terrific position will be a hard act to follow.

Going Out with a Bang

Month 12
Day 30

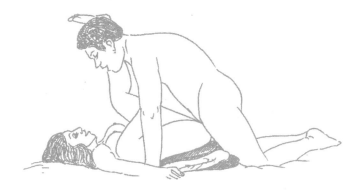

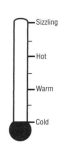

Sizzling

Hot

Warm

Cold

You've made it! It's the last position of the year! You've kept track of all the positions and activities that you've enjoyed this past year, so that you can do them again next year. If you haven't, you'll just have to repeat everything!

For this final position, the woman is on her back. The man is kneeling between the woman's legs. Ladies, rest one leg up on your partner's shoulder. Bend your other leg in front of you so that your foot is on your partner's chest. The closer to your chest you can get your leg, the deeper your partner will be inside of you.

Have your partner slide his penis inside of you as he leans forward. Reach your hand under his stomach so you can masturbate. Let your partner know when you're about to reach your peak so that he can intensify his thrusting. Look him in the eyes as both of you orgasm.

By now your sex life will be spectacular. You're having more sex, and you're having better sex. You will have learned a lot about yourself and your partner this year. Put it to good use for a lifetime of pleasurable experiences.

31 EXTRAS FOR 31-DAY MONTHS

Extra Day 1. January 31: Age of Aquarius

Extra Day 2. March 31: March Madness

Extra Day 3. May 31: Afternoon Delight

Extra Day 4. July 31: A Day to Celebrate

Extra Day 5. August 31: Fun in the Sun

Extra Day 6. October 31: Trick or Treat

Extra Day 7. December 31: Ring in the New Year!

Age of Aquarius

Extra Day 1
January 31

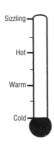

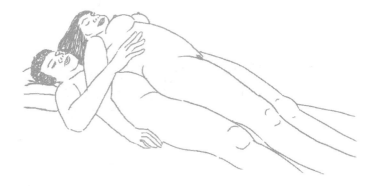

Although today lands in the zodiacal sign Aquarius, everyone can enjoy great sex today. After all, Aquarius is the water bearer and we know great sex needs water and lubrication to keep things slippery and smooth. So no matter what astrological sign you might be, get ready for some fun!

Ladies, your partner needs to lie down on the bed with his legs spread apart. Although you'll eventually be lying down on your partner, this position is much easier to accomplish if you start by sitting up. Facing the same direction as your partner, put your legs in front of you and lower yourself down the shaft of your partner's penis. Once he's securely inside of you, put your legs together to tighten the penetration. Then lean backward all the way to your partner's chest. Use your hand to masturbate.

Guys, with your partner this close to you, there are so many things you can do. Kiss her neck and nibble her ear. Wrap your arms around her and massage her breasts with your hands. Whisper to her. Tell her how wonderful she is and how much you love her. Hold her close while you both climax.

March Madness

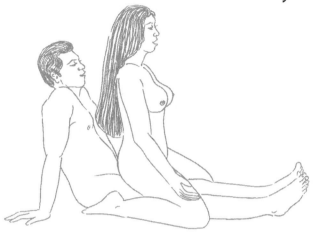

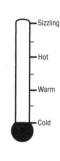

The college basketball champion has been decided, but it's not too late to make a little March madness of your own. You don't need brackets or rankings to make it to the big dance. You just need a willing partner and a love for fun!

For this position, the man sits with his legs straight in front of him. Ladies, sit on your partner's lap facing the same direction he is facing. Bend your legs so that your feet are behind you. Spread your knees apart as wide as possible to make the penetration extra deep for your partner. Use your hand to masturbate while you lift and lower your hips up and down the shaft of your partner's penis.

Guys, put your arms around your partner and hold her close. Use your hands to massage her breasts and stimulate her nipples. Very lightly kiss her on the back of the neck. Most women find this highly arousing. Help her lift and lower her hips until your March madness has been cured.

Afternoon Delight

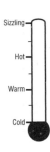

Sizzling
Hot
Warm
Cold

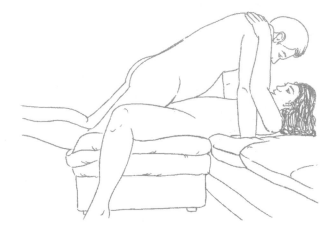

Spring has sprung. The sun is shining bright. And temperatures are rising. It's a great time of year for a playful afternoon of sex.

This position is a variation of the standard missionary position. Instead of having the woman's legs in front of her on the bed, in this position she has her legs straddling a bench or small table. This small modification changes the angle of penetration because the woman's vaginal muscles are pulled downward by her hanging legs. If the woman can reach the floor with her feet, she also has a lot more leverage for thrusting.

One of the biggest benefits of this position is the ability to see your partner's face and make eye contact with them. Guys, stroke your partner's hair and face. Lean forward far enough to kiss her. Rub your chest against her nipples. Both of you can watch your partner's facial expressions as they experience full and deep pleasure.

A Day to Celebrate

Extra Day 4
July 31

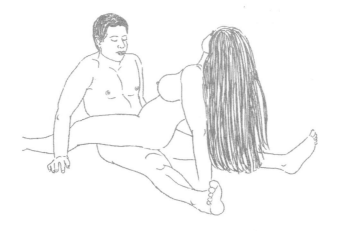

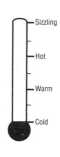

July is Cultivate Your Character Month and National Anti-Boredom Month. Thankfully, it's also National Hot Dog Month, National Ice Cream Month, and National Picnic Month. So pack some hot dogs and ice cream in the picnic basket and find a secluded spot to cultivate your character. If you follow our instructions, you definitely won't be bored!

The man sits with his legs spread wide open. The woman sits on her partner's lap facing him. Ladies, use your hand to guide your partner's hot dog into your picnic basket. Your legs should be over your partner's thighs. Spread them as far apart as you can for the deepest penetration. Then, to make things tight, put your arms behind you and lean backward. A deep,

tight penetration is great for cultivating character!

Let your partner do most of the thrusting. Not only will that help build character, it also reduces the risk of accidentally bending him too far the wrong way. Clench your vaginal muscles together until your partner has filled your cone with ice cream.

Fun in the Sun

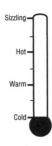

Sizzling

Hot

Warm

Cold

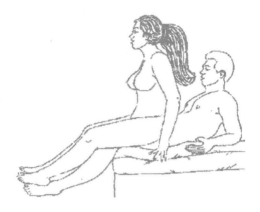

Ah, the good old summertime. It's the hottest season of the year. The days are long and the nights are short. And by now you're nearly ready for the temperatures to cool down, football to start, and fall to arrive. But before you say goodbye to summer, keep the temperatures high with this hot position!

Guys, lie down on the bed with your legs hanging over the edge. Bend your arms behind you so that you're resting on your elbows. This changes the angle of penetration and also gives you a much better view of your partner.

Ladies, sit on your partner's lap facing away from the bed. Keep your legs apart until you've achieved penetration and are sitting comfortably. Then put your legs together on top of your partner's legs for lots of skin-to-skin contact. Although your partner will do most of the thrusting, he won't mind if you lift and lower your hips to meet his.

Guys, use your hands to explore your partner's lower back, hips, and buttocks. Pull your partner's hips to yours for the deepest possible penetration while you orgasm.

Trick or Treat

Extra Day 6
October 31

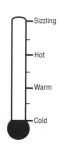

Sizzling

Hot

Warm

Cold

Leave the candy for the kids. You'll be trick-or-treating for something a lot better! So get out your masks and get ready for some Halloween action!

Each of you needs a mask for this intercourse activity. Small ones that just cover the eyes are typically the most comfortable, but also say the least about you (unless, of course, you're a minimalist, in which case it says everything). Try to pick a mask that matches your mood and personality type. Of course, a mask made from a picture of your partner's favorite fantasy person is always popular too.

The idea of this activity is to have fun! It's nearly impossible to be serious when you're having sex wearing a mask and looking at a mask. Many people find that the mask helps them feel less inhibited. Let your wild side show! Use every trick you know to give your partner the best treat you can.

Ring in the New Year!

Extra Day 7

December 31

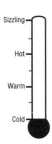

Sizzling
Hot
Warm
Cold

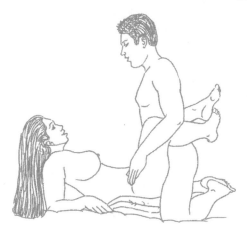

You've decided on your resolutions for next year. You've bought the lucky black-eyed peas for tomorrow's dinner. The champagne is getting cold in the refrigerator. And you've memorized the words to "Auld Lang Syne." It's time to use this position to start celebrating the end of the old and the beginning of the new!

For this position, the woman lies on her back with her arms bent behind her so that she is resting on her elbows. The man is kneeling between the woman's legs, facing her. To make penetration easier, a pillow or two should be placed under the woman's hips.

Guys, put your hands under your partner's buttocks and maneuver her hips to a position where you can easily slide your penis into her vagina. Watch the entrance to her vagina expand as you insert the head. Thrust your hips and watch the shaft sliding in and out. Have your partner wrap her legs around your waist. Not only is this an intimate gesture, it also makes the penetration much deeper. Manually stimulate your partner with your fingers while you thrust. Rub her clitoris back and forth until both of you have peaked.